# Aging Well *with* Cannabis

## Also by Peter Grinspoon

*Free Refills: A Doctor Confronts His Addiction* (2016)

*Seeing Through the Smoke: A Cannabis Specialist Untangles the Truth about Marijuana* (2023)

# Aging Well *with* Cannabis

## *Feel Better, Sleep Better, and Live Better with Marijuana and CBD*

Peter Grinspoon, MD

Foreword by Staci Gruber, PhD, Director, Marijuana Investigations for Neuroscientific Discovery (MIND), McLean Hospital, Harvard Medical School

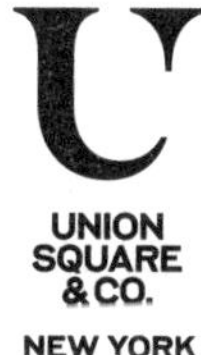

UNION SQUARE & CO.

NEW YORK

*To Emma, Zachary, and Jacob*
*Children are the greatest high of all.*

---



Cover design by Kaylie Pendleton.
Cover image by Shutterstock.com/Irina_iris.


Union Square & Co.
Hachette Book Group
1290 Avenue of the Americas, New York, NY 10104
unionsquareandco.com
@unionsqandco

First Edition: May 2026

Union Square & Co. is an imprint of Grand Central Publishing, a division of Hachette Book Group, Inc. The Union Square & Co. name and logo are registered trademarks of Hachette Book Group, Inc.

The publisher is not responsible for websites (or their content) that are not owned by the publisher.

Union Square & Co. books may be purchased in bulk for business, educational, or promotional use. For information, please contact your local bookseller or the Hachette Book Group Special Markets Department at special.markets@hbgusa.com.

Interior images: Courtesy Getty Images: simpson33 (31), xiao zhou (33), Tinnakorn Jorruang (34), EyeEm Mobile GmbH (156); Shutterstock.com: Mulevich (152); and Stephen Mandile (235).

Print book interior design by Rich Hazelton.

Library of Congress Control Number: 2025050312

ISBNs: 978-1-4549-6293-9 (paperback), 978-1-4549-6294-6 (ebook)

Printed in Canada

MRQ-L

10 9 8 7 6 5 4 3 2 1

# Contents

# Foreword

The Grinspoon legacy is alive and well. In his newest book, *Aging Well with Cannabis*, Dr. Peter Grinspoon once again demonstrates his commitment to an often misunderstood, but absolutely critical area of medicine today.

My first encounter with the Grinspoon family was through Peter's father, Dr. Lester Grinspoon, best known for his pioneering work in cannabis beginning in the 1960s. In a real-life plot twist, Lester embarked on a scientific journey to document the harms of cannabis, but beginning with his friendship with esteemed astrophysicist Carl Sagan, ultimately shifted his perspective—and the rest is history. In 1971, his seminal book, *Marihuana Reconsidered*, reevaluated the existing literature, concluding that cannabis use was not as harmful as the government and medical professionals claimed. Lester's contributions didn't stop there; throughout his sixty-year career as an educator and researcher at Harvard Medical School (HMS), he worked tirelessly to uncover facts about cannabis, not only through eleven books and 180 scientific articles, but also through his advocacy, which helped to shape our current cannabis landscape. In 1993, Lester's *Marihuana: The Forbidden Medicine* served as a key educational resource for doctors and patients, helping to pave the way for California to become the first state to legalize medical cannabis in 1996; the majority of states would eventually follow suit. Although his opinions were highly controversial at the time, Lester's work has influenced every person working in or even adjacent to the cannabis field today—and I am no exception.

Lester's trailblazing efforts undoubtedly made space for my own research, which focuses on identifying and maximizing the potential benefits of medical cannabis and cannabinoid treatments while minimizing risk and harm. As a cognitive neuroscientist at McLean Hospital and an associate professor at HMS, I originally founded a lab dedicated to studying the relationship between symptoms of psychiatric disorders, substance use, and cognition. Like Lester, as I worked on early career projects, including those designed to document potential harms of recreational cannabis use, I also began to see another, often hidden side of the story. While working with patients with bipolar disorder, my curiosity was sparked by stories from many patients who reported that they found cannabis to be extremely helpful in regulating their mood. Patients who were spiraling toward mania found cannabis grounding and stabilizing, while those feeling increasingly depressed or down said it was often uplifting. I could think of no other examples of conventional pharmacotherapy that had a similar impact and needed to know more.

Lester Grinspoon's work was a game-changer and aligned with my belief that cannabinoid-based treatments held extraordinary therapeutic potential for many of these patients, and likely countless others suffering from other conditions. Against the backdrop of rapidly expanding cannabis legalization across the globe, I began exploring the potential therapeutic applications of cannabinoids. In 2014 I launched Marijuana Investigations for Neuroscientific Discovery (MIND), the very first program to assess the long-term impact of medical cannabis use, impossible to envision without Lester's unrelenting efforts.

Today, Dr. Peter Grinspoon continues his family legacy as a primary care physician, devoted to alleviating suffering and promoting health and wellness; he is also fully committed to educating patients, health care providers, and stakeholders about the use of cannabis. He is supremely kind and compassionate, and his work as a medical professional and fierce cannabis advocate serves as a reminder of the importance of empathy—in Peter's case, this actually extends beyond human patients. Not long ago, I came across a stranded juvenile turkey, clearly in need of help, and my first thought was to call Peter and his lovely wife, Liz, for help, as they routinely spend time rescuing and rehabilitating wildlife, offering their home as a sanctuary for animals in need. In typical Grinspoon fashion and without hesitation, they abandoned their afternoon plans and arrived fully outfitted, ready for rescue. Hours later, as darkness fell, we were all still at it, a testament to Peter's unwavering dedication to those in need. His patients often comment on his ability to connect, each feeling seen and heard, a rarity among health care providers today.

Older adults represent the fastest growing group of cannabis consumers across the United States—a fact that many find surprising, but shouldn't. After all, the most common indications for medical cannabis use—chronic pain, anxiety/mood issues, and sleep disruption—are also among the most common complaints across older populations. While an overwhelming majority of Americans support legal access to medical cannabis, health care providers and patients alike often lack information needed to make good decisions regarding cannabis use. Federal and state laws are still discordant, and ongoing debates and legislative efforts surrounding cannabis and hemp can make anyone's head spin. In *Aging Well with Cannabis*, Peter focuses on guiding older adults through the complex world of medical cannabis. As the plant contains more than five hundred compounds, cannabis is not one thing and should never be considered a "one size fits all" solution. So much depends on the reason for use, what products are chosen, and how much, how often, and how it is used. It's also crucial to know what other medications someone is taking, and individual factors like age, metabolism, and genetics must be taken into account. Peter distills many of these complicated issues into a timely, commonsense guide for seniors and their families, who may not know where to start with a complex plant, rife with apparent contradictions. Does cannabis help or harm memory? Worsen or alleviate anxiety? Peter addresses these important questions and many others, forging new ground and creating a novel resource for older adults looking to incorporate cannabis treatment into their lives—and perhaps enjoy their golden years with a little bit of "green."

—Stacy Gruber, MD

# Author's Note

Before we begin, I wish to clarify in advance several points concerning case studies and vignettes, the language used when referring to gender, other potentially stigmatizing language, and issues clarifying the lack of provision of medical advice in this text. Please see below:

**On patients:** All patients represented in case studies and vignettes are composites.

**On gender:** In this book, gender is represented as "he" and "she," for the sake of simplicity, and because virtually all research that has been done on cannabis divides people into those two categories. The author wishes to acknowledge that this may leave out many nonbinary people.

**On language:** The words "cannabis" and "marijuana" are used interchangeably in this book, while historical and racial associations with "marijuana" are acknowledged.

**On medical advice:** None of what is written in these pages should be construed or interpreted as medical advice offered by this author. Always seek guidance from your physician or other qualified health provider regarding the use of cannabis or psychedelic drugs for a specific medical condition or vulnerability.

# Introduction

Our society's views on cannabis are evolving rapidly. As of this writing, medical marijuana has now been legalized in thirty-nine states and the District of Columbia. Many older patients are curious about the ways in which cannabis can help them. Once demonized as a forbidden medicine, cannabis is increasingly being recognized as a natural and relatively nontoxic remedy for such uncomfortable conditions as chronic pain, anxiety, and insomnia. Many of the unpleasant symptoms that accompany the aging process are particularly amenable to treatment with cannabis. Is cannabis right for you? What does and doesn't cannabis treat? How do you get started with cannabis? What are the risks to watch out for? How do we make this process as safe as possible? Read on!

CHAPTER 1

# Cannabis and the Twenty-First Century: Changing Views

Cannabis has tremendous potential to reduce the symptoms and the health-related suffering of seniors—sixty million people in the United States alone. It has great potential to help with common symptoms experienced by aging people, such as anxiety, chronic pain, and insomnia.

However, there have been obstacles to wide adoption of medical cannabis that stem from our country's long-standing war on drugs. As a society, we have prioritized stigmatizing various drugs, including cannabis and psychedelic drugs, over researching how they might be helpful. Consequently, most doctors haven't been taught enough about medical cannabis to know how to advise patients. Misinformation about cannabis is everywhere. When you ask about any issue related to cannabis online, the answers are contradictory. Going to a dispensary can be a bewildering experience. Patients can feel uncomfortable about using a drug that has been so thoroughly stigmatized. It is difficult to obtain clear, practical information about how to use medical marijuana safely and effectively.

Despite those obstacles, older patients represent the demographic in which cannabis use is growing most rapidly, by far. Our elders are seeking symptom relief without relying on a suitcase full of pharmaceuticals. This trend is propelling medical cannabis to the forefront of options for treating their symptoms. Together, with some basic education and with the help of this book, we can make the entire endeavor safer, more effective, and more comfortable.

It may appear as if the use of medical cannabis is a new phenomenon—and a novel component of modern medical practice—as cannabis becomes legal in more and more states. However, humans have used cannabis and hemp since the Neolithic Revolution nearly twelve thousand years ago. That is roughly when *Homo sapiens* transitioned from a hunter-gatherer lifestyle to settled agriculture. Hemp has been with us on our human journey, for medical and spiritual use, since the very beginning of the modern era.

Some of the most ancient human artifacts ever found include a ten-thousand-year-old piece of hemp fabric, discovered in ancient Mesopotamia, and some twelve-thousand-year-old shards of pottery, woven through with hemp cord, that were found in Taiwan. Cannabis has an extensive history as a medicine and a sacrament in many human civilizations. In China, c. 2700 BCE, the mythical emperor Shennong is said to have detailed the medical benefits of cannabis for conditions such as malaria, pain associated with menstruation, and rheumatism. It was also used as an analgesic during childbirth. Cannabis arrived in India c. 2000 BCE and has been used there, in religious rituals, in the form of bhang (a cannabis paste often mixed into a milky drink of the same name), for several millennia. It was also used as an anticonvulsive, a painkiller, an appetite stimulant, and an aphrodisiac—many of the same purposes that we use it for today.

Cannabis was used during the time of the pharaohs (c. 3000 BCE) in Egypt. It was used to treat fevers, to ease urinary and rectal problems, and to help with childbirth. Evidence of cannabis use was also found in Israel, where residues containing THC were discovered in an ancient temple (about 700 BCE). For centuries, cannabis was also used in religious rituals. By 450 BCE, it had made its way to Rome and Greece. Herodotus, the famous Greek historian, wrote about it, as did the legendary physician Galen, who praised cannabis for its ability to relieve earaches and help with relaxation.

During medieval times in Europe, cannabis and hemp extracts were used to help with childbirth, joint pain, convulsions, and toothaches. In the mid-1800s, William O'Shaughnessy, an Irish physician, became convinced of the therapeutic value of cannabis while he was doing medical research in India. Eventually, he popularized the herb's use in England as a remedy for a variety of medical conditions. In describing the merits of cannabis given for acute and chronic rheumatism, O'Shaughnessy claimed that it caused "the alleviation of pain in most, remarkable increase of appetite in all, unequivocal aphrodisia, and great mental cheerfulness."[1] Hemp extracts became a popular medicine during the Victorian era for many of the reasons we use it today—to help with insomnia, menstrual cramps, muscle spasms, and rheumatism.

In the early 1600s, hemp arrived in the American colonies, where it was used industrially. The British needed hemp for sails and ropes for their ships. It wasn't until the 1840s, when the medical community in the United States became aware of William O'Shaughnessy's work, that the potential to use cannabis as a medicine began to gain prominence. In fact, cannabis was widely used as a patent medicine in the United States from the mid- to late 1800s to the early 1900s. In the 1850s, it was listed in the *United States Pharmacopeia*, a compendium of all effective medicines available to physicians. More than a hundred medical articles were published in Western medical journals about medical cannabis, until it was criminalized in 1937.

* * *

The tragic tale of how and why cannabis was criminalized is described in detail in my previous book *Seeing Through the Smoke* (2023). In brief, after Prohibition ended in 1933, a sprawling, resourceful, and avid law enforcement apparatus needed another substance besides alcohol to prohibit. The head of the recently launched Federal Bureau of Narcotics, Harry Anslinger, was an anticannabis zealot who leveraged racism against immigrants from Latin America, associating them, falsely, with cannabis-related crimes. He also exploited racist tropes against Black people, many of whom also used cannabis, to create moral panic about dangerous users of cannabis. Anslinger worked with industrial interests that competed with hemp (e.g., silk, paper) and with media magnate William Randolph Hearst to taint and stigmatize every aspect of cannabis use. In 1937, with the Marijuana Tax Act, it became effectively impossible to prescribe or use cannabis. Several other laws since then have resulted in the arrest of tens of millions of people for simple cannabis possession. Many have been given lengthy prison sentences.

In the early 1970s, President Richard Nixon reinvigorated the nation's war on drugs, although recent tapes[2] have come to light on which he states that cannabis "was not particularly dangerous," a clear indication that Nixon's stance on cannabis, i.e., that it was the nation's "public enemy number one," was completely disingenuous and was politically motivated. Since that time, more than twenty million people have been arrested for nonviolent cannabis possession. Getting arrested for cannabis possession is generally far worse for one's health than using cannabis. A criminal record can undermine one's education, employment, and housing, causing immense stress. There is a racist component to arrest for possession, as well: Although cannabis is used by Black and white people at the same rate, Black people are arrested for it nearly four times as often.[3]

Fortunately, there has also been a strong legalization movement, in which my father, Dr. Lester Grinspoon, played a key role. In 1971, my dad's book *Marihuana Reconsidered*, which discussed the harms and benefits of cannabis in a neutral fashion, was reviewed on the front page of the *New York Times Book Review*. The vast amount of research on marijuana that he synthesized in the book led him to conclude that it should be legalized; he said, "Before we put all our children in jail, let's take an adult look at marihuana." My dad wrote a second book in 1993, *Marihuana: The Forbidden Medicine*, which paved the way for the first state—California—to legalize medical marijuana in 1996.

As of this writing, nonmedical cannabis is fully legal in twenty-five states and decriminalized in seven. More than half of all Americans live in one of those states, where they, as adults, can legally buy and consume cannabis for any reason. Medical marijuana is now legal in the District of Columbia and thirty-nine states—a number that seems to grow with every election cycle. Other states have provisions for the use of CBD and very low levels of THC. It is important to remember that cannabis is still illegal on the federal level, which can make it tricky to travel from state to state with one's supply of medical marijuana.

Around 90 percent of all Americans currently support legal access to medical marijuana, while about 54 percent of Americans, including majorities of Democrats, Republicans, and Independents, support full legalization of recreational and medical marijuana.[4] It is only a matter of time before both medical and recreational marijuana will be fully legal at the federal level. This eventuality will make it much easier for medical marijuana patients, especially those who live in anticannabis states, like Idaho, to treat their conditions with cannabis. In the meantime, it is advisable to be familiar with local and federal laws and to take care not to run afoul of them.

The consequences of the illegality of cannabis have been catastrophic. Today, there is still quite a bit of stigma and disinformation concerning cannabis, as a result of the propagandist war on drugs. Consequently, doctors are behind in their knowledge base. In fact, they are often far behind their own patients. Many physicians don't know enough about marijuana to have helpful conversations about it with their patients or to advise them on how to use it safely and productively. Research into the potential medicinal benefits of cannabis has been delayed for half a century. Most federal funding of research on the topic has been spent on finding harms—and ignoring benefits—to support the societal moral panic needed to wage the war on drugs. Fortunately, all of this is changing, and we are starting to look with curiosity and neutrality into the potential benefits, as well as the harms, of medicinal marijuana.

Even organizations that don't typically stick their necks out are starting to put their support behind medical marijuana, simply because they are unable to ignore the tremendous number of their members who are benefiting from it. Others among them are "canna-curious" and eager to learn if cannabis might be able to help them, too. In a 2019 article, the AARP summarized their position by stating: "The AARP Board of Directors considered the emerging evidence suggesting that marijuana is helpful in treating such conditions and symptoms, then approved a policy supporting the use of medical marijuana in the states that have legalized it."[5]

How radical can it be if the AARP approves medical marijuana? According to a recent study from the AARP, 21 percent of people over the age of fifty have used cannabis. The main reasons they cited for using it were to relax, sleep, feel joy and feel good, relieve pain, improve mood, connect with people, and make social gatherings more fun.[6]

Older patients represent the group in which cannabis use is increasing most rapidly. The rates of use in this population doubled from 2005 to 2015 and roughly doubled once again from 2015 to 2018, up to 4.2 percent.[7] Those numbers might be the result of underreporting, however, as many people in this generation might not feel comfortable admitting to using cannabis, because of lingering stigma. But according to one study of patients over fifty years old, "Attitudes toward cannabis have changed over time with 4 of 5 survey respondents currently holding a favorable attitude."[8]

Seniors are often turned on to cannabis by children or friends. They are discovering that cannabis helps them with many of the symptoms and discomforts of aging and provides more relief than conventional pharmaceuticals—and sometimes with fewer side effects, although cannabis itself isn't entirely free of potentially difficult side effects (see chapter 5 for more information).

As we age, we accumulate diagnoses, specialists, and prescriptions (see chapter 3). "Polypharmacy," the simultaneous use of five or more medications, is common, expensive, confusing, and dangerous. I have many primary care patients who are on ten or more different medications. A few of them are using more than twenty. Older patients are rediscovering that medical marijuana can reduce symptoms, with a relatively low toxicity, if used properly. They are finding that they can reduce their reliance on traditional pharmaceuticals. Many have experienced improved symptom relief, relaxed mood, and a better health-related quality of life, as well as better quality end-of-life care.

Chronic pain, anxiety, and insomnia, among many other symptoms, are epidemic in the sixty-five-and-older crowd. With good intentions, doctors tend to throw medication after medication at these symptoms and ailments. The cost—and side effects—can be additive. In other words, when we prescribe a medication it may alleviate one symptom but aggravate another. For example, we might prescribe a sleeping medication that results in worsened fatigue, balance, and memory. Rarely do we remember to stop, strip off, or pare down medications, let alone "de-prescribe" them. Our medical system is organized for doctors to do more for patients, even though sometimes "less is more." Often, we can help more by doing less and reevaluating treatments that have become unnecessary.

Medical cannabis is fundamentally different from most traditional pharmaceuticals in that it can help treat several symptoms at once. For example, it can help patients with chronic pain, anxiety, and insomnia at the same time. Imagine how many fewer medicines a patient might need to take when medical marijuana comes on board. In addition, studies of medical cannabis consistently show that "health-related quality of life" rises when patients start using medicinal cannabis.[9] Is this not the Holy Grail of most treatments? At the end of the day, our health and the quality of our lives is all we have.

Conventional medical treatments for many conditions, including anxiety, insomnia, and chronic pain, can be particularly toxic to older patients. Take, for example, the case of chronic pain, which afflicts tens of millions of Americans. No doctor wishes to prescribe opioids, no matter how bad the pain is, because they can cause falls, confusion, sedation, constipation, addiction, and delirium—to name just a few problems. NSAIDs (nonsteroidal anti-inflammatory drugs), such as ibuprofen (Advil, Motrin), naproxen (Aleve), or diclofenac (Voltaren) can harm—or even kill—in a variety of ways, including with bleeding, ulcers, heart attacks, and kidney failure. Indeed, we lose approximately sixteen thousand arthritis patients a year from overuse of NSAIDs.[10] Just because a medication is sold over the counter doesn't mean it is safe! Acetaminophen (Tylenol) doesn't do much in the way of relieving chronic pain, and it can harm your liver. Likewise, the drug gabapentin (Neurontin), which is frequently prescribed to alleviate chronic pain, has a very modest benefit, but can make a patient feel brain-fogged and exhausted. All of those medications are more dangerous for older patients than they are for younger patients.

Older patients are discovering that while cannabis can help alleviate symptoms of chronic pain, it might also have a pleasant and helpful effect on their mood. This is especially true if cannabis is dosed properly—it is imperative to not take too much at first, to "start low and go slow." Taking a dose of cannabis that is too high can be a miserable experience and can even be dangerous. The right dose for people can vary widely. So it is important to take the time you need to get up to speed on medical cannabis. Work with your doctor or with an informed cannabis specialist. Keep in mind that there are some flakes out there, as in any field, so it is important to do your research or get a good referral from a source you trust. Start with an extremely low dose and slowly inch the dosage upward until the desired effect is reached.

As more science substantiates the medicinal benefits of cannabis, increasing numbers of seniors are using medical cannabis.

Many of them are first introduced to it by their children, who have experienced medicinal benefits from cannabis and wish to share it with their parents. Unfortunately, the kids don't always recommend a low enough dose to start with, since they might require a much higher dose for themselves.

Recent studies show a dramatic increase in symptom relief from cannabis in older populations, with relatively infrequent and mild side effects. In one 2018 study, "Epidemiological Characteristics, Safety and Efficacy of Medical Cannabis in the Elderly," Israeli researchers studied 2,736 medical cannabis patients who were sixty-five years of age or older. They found that a large majority of patients responded positively.

> After six months of treatment, 93.7 percent of the respondents reported improvement in their condition, and the reported pain level was reduced from a median of 8 on a scale of 0–10 to a median of 4. Most common adverse events were dizziness (9.7 percent) and dry mouth (7.1 percent). After six months, 18.1 percent stopped using opioid analgesics or reduced their dose.[11]

These findings are consistent with my own clinical experiences with treating older adults with cannabis.

Having said that, cannabis is not for everyone. Some people have bad reactions, such as anxiety or dizziness. Other patients have fallen down or fainted, while still others have medical conditions that make cannabis use even more dangerous. Some just don't like the feeling or find that it makes them too sleepy. And, as with all drugs and medications, cannabis doesn't work for all people. When it does work, it can be transformative.

## JUDITH

Judith is a spry ninety-three-year-old, who is active and mentally clear at baseline. Each day, she walks farther than most twenty-year-olds. She started having severe upper back and neck pain, which was keeping her up at night. I advised her to see her primary care doctor to make sure that nothing serious was going on and to purchase an ergonomic pillow. She was diagnosed with arthritis. Because Judith was on a blood thinner, she couldn't take NSAIDs, and she didn't wish to get a steroid injection. She was afraid to try opioids due to noxious side effects, which included falls and constipation. Tylenol didn't have the slightest impact on her pain. Her doctor tried Tylenol with a small dose of codeine, and also tried gabapentin. Although those medications succeeded in blunting Judith's symptoms, they also saddled her with unpleasant side effects, such as excessive daytime fatigue and constipation.

I started Judith on one-half of a 5-milligram gummy, a mere 2.5 milligrams of THC. For context, one puff of today's strong marijuana contains about 5–10 milligrams of THC. I reminded Judith that it would take forty-five to ninety minutes to absorb the gummy and feel the effects. I warned her not to take a second dose that evening. I didn't want her to make the rookie mistake of taking a second dose of an edible before the first one kicks in, because that can make you feel unpleasantly and overly intoxicated. I nag patients about this all the time, as I don't want them to take too large a dose, have a bad outcome, and then be turned off from the entire endeavor. If you wish to increase the dose of your edible, it is best to do so the next day, not thirty minutes after taking the first dose, because it can take up to ninety minutes to be fully absorbed.

When purchasing gummies, or if your kids provide them, please confirm the dosage before consuming them, and confirm that they are, in fact, the dose you are expecting. You do not want to take too much. Standard gummies contain 5 milligrams, which is in the right vicinity of the dosage you'd want to start with, although I often have people start with half of one gummy, 2.5 milligrams. Marijuana dispensaries sell much stronger gummies, so it is imperative to confirm the dose before purchasing them. Avoid homemade edibles, especially if you aren't absolutely clear on the dose.

With the gummy, Judith's back and neck pain was completely alleviated. She could wake up without pain, enjoy yoga, and walk around without suffering. As for side effects, she said, "I haven't slept this well since I was a teenager, and I wake up in such a good mood." She no longer needs Tylenol with codeine or the gabapentin that her doctor gave her—which were unpleasant to take. Judith's back pain got somewhat better with physical therapy and, as time went on, she only needed to use one gummy about three times per week, which was an improvement for her pocketbook. Judith had no negative side effects from the gummy and reported being mentally clear upon awakening.

---

There are many unfortunate obstacles that keep older patients from the benefits of using medical cannabis. For example, internet searches for anything related to cannabis offer "answers" that are flatly contradictory: It harms memory. It helps with memory. You gain weight. You lose weight. It helps nausea. It causes vomiting. Which is true? To make things worse, most information about cannabis is presented from a very one-sided "pro" or "anti" vantage point, depending on the biases and personal beliefs of the particular expert. We need a balanced consideration of cannabis, without idealizing its benefits or minimizing—or wildly exaggerating—its harms.

Educating people about the potential harms of cannabis (see chapter 5) is just as important as teaching them about the benefits. Soaring enthusiasm for treatments can transcend the actual scientific evidence. Advertising claims can be exceedingly misleading. For example, anyone who suggests that cannabis "cures" cancer or Covid is misguided. It doesn't. Cannabis has plenty of known harms, which we can usually manage and minimize with education and regulation. The essential concerns are that cannabis should be avoided by teenagers and pregnant or breastfeeding women, as well as by patients with a history or family history of psychotic diseases, such as bipolar disorder or schizophrenia. Cardiac patients should use it with extreme caution.

Older patients have aged out of many of those concerns. They are past the window for developing a primary psychotic disorder and they can't get pregnant. For those who are older, there are different things to watch out for, however, when starting medicinal cannabis. It's essential to pay particular attention to the acute impairment that can affect the cannabis novice, especially until they get used to the effects. Of concern are potential falls, temporary memory impairment, and confusion. Patients with cardiac conditions, such as arrythmias or coronary disease, need to proceed with extreme caution, keep the dosages of cannabis low, and avoid smoking it altogether. As with all human endeavors, knowledge is power and, in this case, knowledge results in safety and efficacy.

If you, or a loved one, wish to explore the possibility of using medical cannabis to help alleviate some of your symptoms, this book is for you. You will learn which conditions cannabis can and cannot help, and how you can safely get started on cannabis.

## Top 11 Myths About the Use of Medical Cannabis

These are the objections to the use of medical cannabis that I have heard from various colleagues over the years. Although they lessen over time, they still persist.

**Myth #1:** People smoke medical marijuana, which means it isn't a safe medicine.
**Reality:** A friend of mine, a psychiatrist, once yelled at me, "How can a burning plant be considered a medicine?" There are numerous ways to consume cannabis that are safer than smoking it. These include ingestible forms, such as edibles and tinctures, which are not harmful to the lungs, and which allow for careful control of dosing. Most of the harms of cannabis that have been demonstrated were based on studies of smoked cannabis. There is much less evidence that edibles and tinctures (see chapter 2) are dangerous. As with other drugs and medications, there are safe and less safe ways to use cannabis, and smoking it is clearly less safe than other consumption methods.

**Myth #2:** There is no evidence that cannabis is an effective medication.
**Reality:** Currently, there is an abundance of evidence that cannabis helps with conditions such as chronic pain, anxiety, insomnia, nausea, muscle spasm in MS (multiple sclerosis), and many other conditions (see chapter 4). Cannabis doesn't treat everything effectively, as some advocates believe, but it is simply not true that there isn't evidence that cannabis is an effective medication for many conditions. In fact, the evidence base grows every day.

**Myth #3:** Cannabis is as addictive as alcohol.
**Reality:** Cannabis certainly can be addictive (see chapter 5), but it is less addictive than alcohol, stimulants, benzodiazepines, opioids, and tobacco. Although an addiction to cannabis can be incredibly destructive, it isn't as dangerous as alcohol or opioid addiction, generally because it isn't life-threatening. Cannabis is about as addictive as coffee—which is not insignificant.

**Myth #4:** Cannabis lowers IQ.
**Reality:** Initial studies, conducted during the war on drugs, appeared, at first glance, to demonstrate a drop in IQ in teens. These studies received a lot of media attention. When the data was reevaluated and socioeconomic factors (e.g., poverty, educational attainment) were accounted for, they showed that there was absolutely no drop in IQ.[12] What the research came down to is that poor, disadvantaged kids, who tend to use cannabis more, are more likely to do worse on standardized tests than more affluent kids. In sum, cannabis does not cause a low IQ.

**Myth #5:** Cannabis lowers motivation.
**Reality:** Cannabis doesn't lower motivation. This myth was spread by the widely criticized DARE (Drug Abuse Resistance Education) program that was used, unsuccessfully, to scare people away from cannabis and other drugs. Because depressed or disadvantaged people sometimes use cannabis to blunt their pain, it can look like their motivation is being sapped by it. Some of the most motivated people throughout history—scientists, musicians, writers, artists—have used cannabis, providing strong evidence that cannabis *can* contribute to motivation.

**Myth #6:** Cannabis causes cancer.

**Reality:** Smoking cannabis is clearly not healthy for the heart or the lungs, as the smoke contains unhealthy combustion products. Yet cannabis has not been linked with lung cancer or emphysema/COPD (chronic obstructive pulmonary disease). However, smoking cannabis can irritate the lungs, causing chronic bronchitis, and can temporarily worsen asthma. Cannabis taken through *other* modes, such as tinctures and edibles, is not linked with lung problems. It is still possible that cannabis may be linked to lung cancer at some point in the future, which is why we advise people not to smoke it.

A possible exception might be the very weak link between cannabis use and both testicular and head and neck cancers.[13] If that link is shown to be true, it will likely prove that the cancer is a result of smoking cannabis, rather than of the use of cannabis itself.

**Myth #7:** A positive drug test means you are intoxicated.

**Reality:** This comes up commonly in preemployment drug screens or after auto accidents. Cannabis is fat soluble, which means that it sticks around in our fat cells, and can be detected in urine for weeks, or even months, after use. A positive test generally means that a person has used cannabis within the last several weeks. It does not mean that they are acutely intoxicated, or even that they were intoxicated within the last day or two. In this respect, cannabis is totally different from alcohol, where the level of alcohol in the blood directly correlates with the level of intoxication.

**Myth #8:** Cannabis causes schizophrenia.

**Reality:** Cannabis can trigger severe psychosis, most commonly in teens and young adults (see chapter 5), although it is rare. Cannabis might also precipitate symptoms of schizophrenia earlier in people who are genetically prone to develop schizophrenia than it would in the general population. That effect of cannabis is a particular concern because the longer one can delay the onset of schizophrenia, the more "adult" life skills can be learned, and the more independent and functional a person can be. However, cannabis doesn't "cause" schizophrenia. We know that because the rates of schizophrenia have been relatively stable worldwide over the last seventy years, while the number of cannabis users has gone up 1,000-fold during the same time frame.[14] If cannabis "caused" schizophrenia, we would have seen a vast increase in the number of cases of schizophrenia, which has not happened.

**Myth #9:** Using cannabis affects your cognitive function.
**Reality:** The data has been confusing over the years. Cannabis use does not permanently harm your memory, except possibly in young teenagers who use a ton of it—although the data on this is inconclusive. Cannabis is known to cause a transient decrement in short-term memory, which also contributes to the stoner stereotype. This effect fully resolves after a few hours. On the other hand, some studies[15] of medical cannabis patients show that cognitive functioning significantly improved, across several domains, after the patients started using medical marijuana. There are many theories as to why this improvement was observed for medical patients but not for recreational marijuana patients. One likely explanation is that when sleep and pain are better controlled, cognitive functioning improves.

Cannabis has been used as an aid to creativity for thousands of years. It enhances the functioning of certain parts of your brain, while temporarily stifling others. Many find it to be an intellectual stimulant. Work by Dr. Staci Gruber at Harvard Medical School's McLean Hospital has shown an improvement in cognitive function among medical cannabis users (see pages 106–107).

**Myth #10:** Cannabis makes you sterile.
**Reality:** Cannabis has not been shown to cause a clinically meaningful effect on virility or fertility. Some data shows that it might affect sperm count. While the evidence is contradictory, some studies have shown that heavy use of cannabis can affect the number of sperm, their movement, and their shape. This has not translated into any measurable effects on fertility or the health of the future children.[16]

**Myth #11:** Cannabis makes you gain weight or become overweight.
**Reality:** Cannabis helps with nausea and poor appetite by giving people the munchies. People may eat more under the influence of cannabis, it's true, yet chronic users tend to weigh less, not more. That might be because they are more active, or because they become tolerant to some of the effects of cannabis.

CHAPTER 2

# What Is Cannabis and How Is It Used?

Cannabis is a complex plant that contains more than five hundred different chemicals, many of which contribute to its medicinal and recreational effects. That is why different types or "strains" (or, as scientists call them, "chemovars") of cannabis can have different effects. Some types might make you feel drowsy and relaxed, whereas others can be more energizing and uplifting. It is often a process of trial and error to find the specific cannabis product that will help alleviate your symptoms. In chapter 6, I discuss how some of the differences between strains—and the marketing claims around them—are exaggerated and how to wade through the hype to get what you need.

The main ingredient in marijuana is tetrahydrocannabinol or, simply, THC. THC is what makes people feel "high" when they use cannabis. Some people love the gentle euphoria and relaxation of a high, while others find it disorienting and annoying. By controlling the amount of THC and using a combination of other components in cannabis, however, people can often attain symptom control while avoiding side effects that they don't like.

Cannabidiol, or CBD, is another main ingredient in cannabis. CBD has been growing in popularity. (See chapter 7 for a more thorough discussion of CBD.) CBD doesn't make people high or impair them in any way, which means it can be safer and more convenient for daytime use, and it can be taken before going to work or driving a car. CBD is often used for conditions such as chronic pain, anxiety, and insomnia, and it is an FDA-approved medication (Epidiolex) for various childhood epilepsy syndromes. CBD is also a strong anti-inflammatory that can help people who are experiencing pain and inflammation and who can't take NSAIDs for medical reasons. There is growing interest in the potential use of CBD for other indications, for example, to help treat addiction, autism, or, as a medicine, psychosis.

THC and CBD, and many other molecules in the cannabis plant, are called "cannabinoids" because they work on our body's ECS (endocannabinoid system). The ECS is one of our most important neurotransmitter systems. It comprises a constellation of neurotransmitters and receptors that are located in the brain and throughout the body. The ECS controls a host of bodily functions, such as appetite, memory, learning, and reproduction. The ECS is what keeps our bodies in homeostasis, or in balance, by managing the levels of other neurotransmitter systems in the body. All of us produce natural cannabis-like molecules called endocannabinoids, which, along with two cannabinoid receptors (CB1 and CB2), form the endocannabinoid system. Cannabis triggers those receptors, and it is largely through the ECS that cannabis works its effects.

There are about a hundred other cannabinoids in the cannabis plant beyond THC and CBD. Many of them will likely have medical potential, once they have been isolated and fully studied. You may have heard of some of these molecules, which are being manufactured and marketed. Often, marketing claims about them are not supported by science, however, as this industry is completely unregulated—a big problem when it comes to quality control. You may have heard about these cannabinoids (described in more detail on pages 197–198):

- **CBN (cannabinol):** Used for sleep; often used with THC or CBD
- **CBG (cannabigerol):** Used for muscle pain, anxiety, colitis, and to stimulate appetite
- **CBC (cannabichromene):** Helpful for pain and as an anti-inflammatory
- **THCV (tetrahydrocannabivarin):** Helps control appetite and blood sugar
- **CBDA (acidic version of CBD):** A very strong anti-inflammatory that helps relieve muscle and nerve pain

In addition to cannabinoids, the marijuana plant has molecules called "terpenes" that contribute to its distinctive smell and taste. It's also likely that terpenes contribute to the psychoactive effect and medicinal benefit of marijuana, although we are still disentangling the exact effects of terpenes.

These are a few of the major terpenes:

- **Myrcene:** Thought to be an analgesic and can have a sedative effect. It is also found in mangos.
- **Limonene:** Has antidepressive, anti-anxiety, and anti-inflammatory properties. Limonene is found in lemons and limes.
- **Pinene:** Thought to alleviate some of the short-term memory impairment that comes with use of THC. When people "bathe" in pine forests, they enjoy breathing in the scent of pinene.
- **β-caryophyllene:** Helps as an anti-inflammatory, with anxiety, and as a painkiller. Black pepper, cloves, and hops have β-caryophyllene.
- **Linalool:** Helps with mood and anxiety and is an anti-inflammatory. It is found in lavender.

## PRESCRIPTION CANNABIS MEDICINES

In addition to the FDA-approved, CBD-based medicine Epidiolex, which is prescribed for childhood epilepsy syndromes, there are several other cannabis-based medicines that have been approved for medical use in the US and Europe.

- **Marinol** and **Syndros** both contain dronabinol, which is a synthetic version of delta-9-THC, the active ingredient in cannabis. Few patients who use these products say they are as effective as regular cannabis. This is likely because they have only THC and not the other molecules that contribute to the medicinal benefit, such as the other, minor cannabinoids and terpenes.
- **Cesamet,** chemical name nabilone, is a synthetic chemical with a pharmacological action similar to that of THC. It is approved in the US for CINV (chemotherapy-induced nausea and vomiting) in patients who have been failed by conventional treatments. Though effective, it tends to have worse side effects than regular cannabis.
- **Sativex,** or the generic nabiximols, is a plant-based extract containing equal amounts of THC and CBD and can be sprayed into the mouth. The spray is legal in dozens of countries (but, sadly, not in the US) for treatment of MS-related spasticity and other conditions. There is very good data demonstrating its efficacy.

## OTHER CBD PRODUCTS

There are many other CBD products on sale that range from the fun to the ridiculous. On the fun side, there are CBD bath bombs, which can be extremely relaxing. On the ridiculous side, there are pillowcases, bras, and workout clothing that are supposedly impregnated with CBD, and that are marketed to help relieve pain and inflammation. This is all nonsense, and it just goes to show how unregulated this industry is if they can make such outrageous claims about anything and everything.

Some coffee shops will even give you the option of getting a shot of CBD with your coffee, for some extra relaxation or an extra boost. I am not a fan of this, as it is impossible to know what exactly, and how much CBD, they are giving you. Is it a safe and regulated product free of THC and other contaminants? If you don't know what you're getting, stick to the medicinal CBD you have bought, which is a known quantity.

There are products on the market that have very high ratios of CBD to THC, and that are helpful for many conditions. If you are trying to avoid impairment, however, you must use caution. Just because there is a high ratio of CBD to THC in a product, it doesn't mean there isn't enough THC to be harmful. Even with a very high ratio of 25:1 CBD:THC you can easily consume enough THC to become impaired. For example, if you take one gummy with 100 milligrams of CBD and 4 milligrams of THC (a 25:1 ratio), know that 4 milligrams of THC is certainly enough for most people to feel a psychoactive effect. Even though 4 milligrams is a relatively low dose (for comparison, one puff of cannabis is 5–10 milligrams of THC), I would never drive after taking 4 milligrams of THC.

## HEMP-DERIVED PRODUCTS

It is important to mention the newly ubiquitous hemp-derived products, which, as the name implies, are derived from the hemp plant. The only difference between cannabis or marijuana and hemp is the amount of THC in the plant. Hemp plants, by law, are less than 0.3 percent THC—not enough to meaningfully cause impairment—in contrast to cannabis/marijuana, which contains upward of 20 percent THC, and can be purchased in a dispensary.

Hemp products became legal when the 2018 US Farm Bill, which included the Hemp Farming Act, legalized hemp production. This bill stipulated that any products that can be derived chemically from the CBD contained in hemp are legal. According to the law of unintended consequences, the Farm Bill didn't anticipate the arrival of a host of new psychoactive products that would be legalized and made widely available.

Hemp-derived products are popping up everywhere—on the internet, in smoke shops, and even at gas stations. Unfortunately, there is absolutely no regulatory framework for these products, which means that they have not been tested. What's worse, it is easy for teens to get their hands on these products—the use of which boils down to a huge, uncontrolled experiment on their vulnerable brain cells. It is no wonder that various states are outlawing them. But that isn't necessarily the right solution because products like these end up on the illicit market and are even more dangerous. They are often of very poor quality, have misleading labels, and represent a menace to public health. Generally, they should be avoided, though many of the low-THC products containing CBD are ethically made and people are using them with good benefit. These products, some of which are described here, can look exactly like regular cannabis products, so . . . buyer beware!

- **Delta-8 THC:** This is popularly described as the mellow version of cannabis, or "THC light." The reality is that when you order Delta-8 on the internet or buy it in a smoke shop, you don't have any idea what you are getting, and the products are often contaminated with dangerous industrial reactants. Even if you manage to get actual Delta-8 THC, you should know that none of the claims about it have been proven.

- **Delta-10 THC:** Another type of THC that is chemically similar to the chief active ingredient in cannabis, Delta-9, Delta-10 THC is found in cannabis but, like so many other hemp products, it hasn't been thoroughly tested in humans.
- **HHC:** A newly developed, highly psychoactive synthetic cannabinoid that hasn't been studied yet (for more on synthetic cannabinoids, see the section below); I would avoid HHC at all costs, as people can overdose and have toxic reactions to it.
- **THC-O:** This is a strong synthetic cannabinoid, several times stronger than regular THC from cannabis, which, supposedly, has more of a "psychedelic effect." THC-O is new and completely untested in humans. Some people who are using it have panic attacks and end up in the ER. It is strongly advised to avoid THC-O.

## SYNTHETIC CANNABINOIDS

Finally, for the sake of completeness, a word about the synthetic cannabinoids that one hears about on the news. These dangerous chemicals are readily available on the internet, and are sold under the common names of K2, spice, and bath salts (which aren't used for baths—they are just sold as "bath salts" to get around the laws that restrict them). The synthetic molecules in these substances trigger the endocannabinoid system in a way that is massive, uncontrolled, and potentially life-threatening. Synthetic cannabinoids, which are frequently used by teenagers, can cause severe psychosis and seizures. A few of the newer synthetic cannabinoids, including recently discovered molecules such as HHC and THCP, have been legalized because they can be derived from hemp. But these products are exceedingly dangerous. If you are interested in stimulating your endocannabinoid system for medical or recreational purposes, stick to cannabis.

## DIFFERENT WAYS TO CONSUME CANNABIS

This section will go over the most common ways to consume cannabis: smoking, vaping, using a tincture under the tongue, eating some type of edible (including chocolate, gummies, pills, and seltzers), using topicals, and using suppositories, and what the benefits and drawbacks are of each.

### Smoking

Most doctors don't recommend smoking cannabis. Smoking involves incinerating the cannabis flower and then inhaling unhealthy combustion products, such as tar, benzene, and carbon monoxide. Inhaled carbon monoxide is thought to contribute to cardiovascular disease, regardless of whether it comes from a cigarette or a joint. However, smoking is a common way to consume cannabis recreationally, say at a party.

To put things into perspective, it is likely that smoking cannabis will not be particularly bad for you if you are an adult who smokes occasionally and modestly—a few puffs on the weekend, for example. Medical patients often require a steady, regular dose of cannabis, especially those who need to use it every day. For these patients, smoking cannabis can cause as many problems as it may alleviate. Most patients would be much better off with other methods of consumption, such as ingesting tinctures and edibles.

One reason cannabis users frequently choose to smoke is that it results in near-instantaneous symptom reduction. Another advantage is that smoking allows for precise dose titration, which means that you can quickly figure out the right dose for yourself, without overshooting. Because cannabis acts so rapidly when it is smoked, you can easily know, within seconds to minutes, if you've taken enough or if you need more. It is very easy to get to the right level.

A downside of smoking cannabis, however, aside from damaging your lungs, is that it gives relief for only a few hours at a time. Other forms, such as edibles or tinctures, provide longer relief. If pain or anxiety is troubling you around the clock, or if you tend to wake up in the middle of the night with insomnia, longer-acting cannabis preparations that last for more than a couple of hours would be more helpful.

There are certain circumstances in which smoking cannabis might be a reasonable medical option. For example, for someone who is dying of cancer, smoking might be a convenient way to immediately get relief from pain or nausea. My brother Danny passed away from leukemia at age sixteen, and for him, smoking cannabis was invaluable in helping to maintain his weight and mood. If you are dying of cancer, or from another end-stage illness, you won't be too worried about what your lungs will look like in twenty to thirty years. Under those circumstances, it makes sense to keep patients as comfortable as possible and use whatever method is most effective for them.

Another exception to the "you shouldn't smoke cannabis" rule applies to people who are on chemotherapy and need rapid relief from nausea. That is what smoking provides, and why it is a common delivery technique for cancer patients. Taking an edible doesn't cut it in that scenario, unless you're consuming them around the clock. A patient might still need a puff or two if they feel the urgency to vomit. Also, if you are undergoing chemo, you might not feel like eating an edible, or anything else, for that matter.

It is of course up to the individual to decide whether or not they wish to assume the risks of smoking cannabis versus using another consumption method. No one should be judged or shamed, beyond receiving a well-intentioned reminder from their doctor, if they choose to smoke cannabis, even if it is not the safest consumption method. Nevertheless, one should not expose others to secondhand smoke. To put this in perspective, smoking cannabis is not as harmful as smoking cigarettes, and it has not been linked with the development of lung cancer or any deaths.[1]

If you decide to smoke cannabis, you can roll a joint; smoke a prerolled joint purchased at a dispensary (which is easier than rolling your own, but more expensive); or use a pipe. The best option is a dry herb vaporizer (see below), which heats up the cannabis but doesn't fully burn it. If you choose to smoke, start with the tiniest inhalation to avoid coughing and prevent accidental overconsumption. Cannabis flower is incredibly strong these days compared to what you may have smoked in college. After your first puff, you can wait a few minutes and then try a second inhalation in order to slowly work your way up to the proper dosage. I strongly suggest that you avoid smoking *anything*, if you have COPD or emphysema, or heart disease. If you have asthma, approach smoking cannabis with caution and make sure that it doesn't trigger wheezing or bronchospasm.

## Vaping

"Vaping" is a term that is used, synonymously, for two separate methods of inhaling cannabis, and that confuses everyone. Fortunately, there is a simple distinction between the two types of vaping: a dry herb vaporizer, which heats up the cannabis flower, and a vape pen, in which synthetic oils are heated. As you might have guessed, the first means of inhaling cannabis is far safer than the second.

### *Dry Herb Vaporizer (the safest inhalation technique)*

A dry herb vaporizer provides the medicinal benefits and convenience of inhalation, but has few of the drawbacks, since it works instantaneously, and it is easy to titrate the dose. The vaporizer heats up the cannabis just enough to produce a vapor (not smoke), but not enough to burn or incinerate the cannabis flower. Consequently, the vapor contains fewer of the toxic combustion products that are found in cannabis smoke, and this method is likely less unhealthy than using a vape pen—although it is somewhat less discreet and less convenient.

It costs a couple hundred dollars to purchase a dry herb vaporizer. To use it, you need to grind cannabis flower in a grinder, a small device that you can easily purchase at any dispensary or smoke shop. Then you put the ground cannabis into a small compartment or well in the center of the vaporizer. Next, you press a button, which causes the device to heat the cannabis in the well. In about fifteen to thirty seconds, it heats the cannabis to 350°F–400°F (177°C–204°C), a temperature that is high enough to vaporize the medicinal components, but not high enough to burn or incinerate the cannabis into smoke.

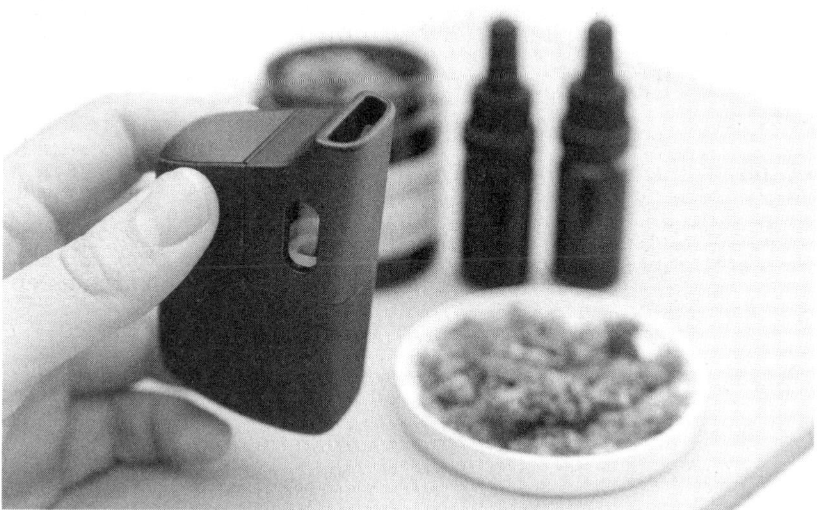

**An example of a dry herb vaporizer, which presents a potentially safer method of inhaling cannabis.**

People quickly get used to using a dry herb vaporizer, even though it involves a few more steps than simply smoking. The user must fill the vaporizer and wait for it to heat up, all of which can be accomplished in a minute or two. In addition to being safer and easier on the lungs, using a dry herb vaporizer is much more cost-effective. That's because it is a closed system, and you don't lose half of the flower in the form of smoke that wafts away. The same amount of cannabis goes a lot further with this method of consumption. When you inhale from a dry herb vaporizer, it tastes much better, too, because instead of inhaling smoke, you are inhaling a vapor of flavorful cannabinoids. Burning can destroy the terpenes that give cannabis its smell and flavor, but they remain intact with a dry herb vaporizer, resulting in a much more pleasurable experience.

Dry herb vaping is almost always what I recommend to patients who wish to inhale cannabis. In my experience, dry herb vaporizers are easier on the lungs than smoking or using a vape pen, and they also allow you to taste the different, delicate flavors of cannabis which, for some people, is a large component of their enjoyment.

Dry herb vaporizers are more economical than smoking, too, because they are self-contained, which means you don't lose most of the product to smoke that just wafts away. Although we need more data on the long-term effects of using dry herb vaporizers, they certainly seem to be the safest option for inhaling cannabinoids at this point.

#### *Vape Pen (convenient, but less safe than a dry herb vaporizer)*

A vape pen is a small device that heats cannabis-impregnated oils until they produce a type of vapor/smoke that is inhaled. Shaped like a pen, it can discreetly fit into your pocket. It emits very little smoke and is a lot less smelly and attention-grabbing than smoking cannabis. You can buy one from a dispensary, as a "pen" or a "vape pen."

They are incredibly simple to use. All you need to do is press a button and inhale, while some vape pens are activated simply by inhaling.

Vape cartridges comprise different types or strains, and they are often divided into indica, sativa, or hybrid (see page 69). You can buy a disposable vape pen or one with a rechargeable battery. If the vape pen is reusable, all you have to do is replace the cartridge that contains the cannabis oil when it is empty. Each cartridge gives you about two hundred to three hundred puffs, so they last a while, unless you consume a heavy amount of cannabis. Vape pens are an extremely convenient way to consume cannabis, and they don't create much of a smell or attract much attention. It doesn't look like you are consuming weed when you use one of these pens, because puffing from a tobacco vape looks the same.

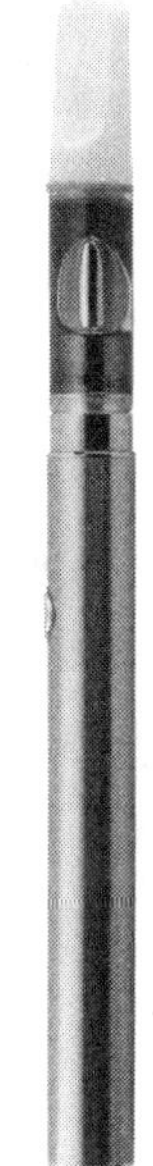

**Vape pens are quite discreet and can easily fit into a pocket. They can be very useful for a patient who is out in public and needs to take a quick, surreptitious puff to avoid vomiting from the side effects of chemotherapy.**

When you first start using a vape pen, be careful not to take a humongous dose on your first puff until you get used to using the apparatus. You might end up gasping for air and feel way too stoned. Personally, I am not a fan of these pens, as I find them to be exceedingly harsh on the lungs. Vape pens trigger my asthma, which doesn't happen when I use a dry herb vaporizer. The industry that produces them is barely regulated. These vapes contain God-knows-what chemicals in the oils, and often are made of dodgy metals that might leach into the oil from the apparatus. Many people are tempted to buy less expensive, poorer quality vapes on the illicit market, but they are even less safe than those you can buy legally. That's how we stumbled on the EVALI (e-cigarette or vaping product-use associated lung injury) crisis that sickened so many people in 2019, although the culprits in that case were mostly illegal nicotine vapes.

### *Metered-Dose Inhalers*

As another inhalation option, people can get metered-dose inhalers—which are just like asthma inhalers—from some dispensaries. These devices allow you to inhale cannabis without any smoke or vapor, which is a convenient and safe way to consume cannabinoids, and they are designed to be less irritating to the lungs than smoking is.

## Tinctures

Tinctures are, in my opinion, one of the best ways to use cannabis. A patient can put as little as a drop or two under their tongue, depending on what dose they want. One must keep it there for a minute or two so that it can fully absorb under the tongue, where there are a lot of blood vessels, making it ideal for absorption. This method works quickly, within twenty to thirty minutes.

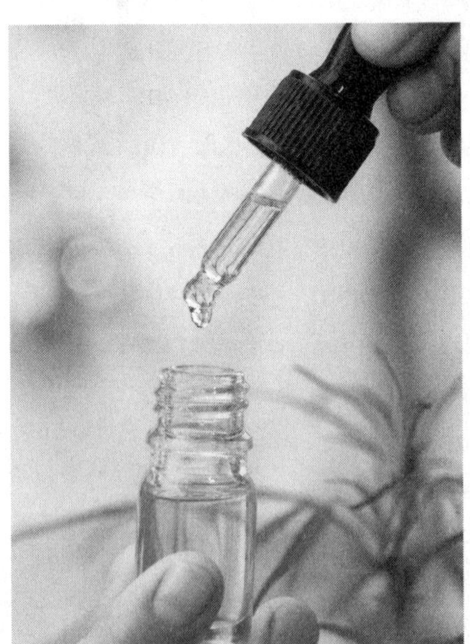

**Tinctures are a nice compromise between the quick convenience of inhaling and the long-lasting effects of edibles. They can also be added to a beverage, such as a relaxing herb tea, at night.**

Although it is a slower method than inhaling cannabis, which works almost immediately, tinctures kick in much more quickly than traditional edibles, such as gummies or chocolate, which can take forty-five to ninety minutes to take effect.

Because tinctures are dispensed in a graduated dropper, it is easy to titrate and control your dose, and to slowly work your way up on the medication. You only need to read how many milligrams are in each dropperful and do some simple math. For example, if there are 10 milligrams of THC per dropperful, and you want to take only 2.5 milligrams, then you simply take one-quarter of a dropperful. Unfortunately, the various products and droppers that you will encounter in dispensaries aren't standardized yet. They will be, eventually, when cannabis is fully legalized and regulated on the federal level. For now, you must look carefully at each tincture bottle for specific concentrations so that you can do the math and figure out your dosage.

If you wish to start at a very low dose of THC, such as 1 or 2 milligrams, as many older patients do, this is most easily done with a tincture. Using a dropper is easier than trying to cut or bite off one-fifth or two-fifths of a 5-milligram gummy. Instead, you simply take the calculated number of drops. If you don't like the taste or feel of it under your tongue, you can put a few drops of tincture into your beverage at night, although then it would absorb as slowly as an edible.

Another advantage of tinctures is that they frequently contain a variety of different cannabis components, such as CBD and other cannabinoids. I generally have patients use at least some CBD with THC because the two elements work well together to help alleviate most symptoms. CBD is also thought to help protect against some of the side effects of THC, such as short-term memory impairment (see chapter 7 for more about

CBD). Instead of buying CBD and THC separately, you can purchase a bottle that contains both. For example, I might start a patient on a tincture with a 4:1 ratio of CBD to THC, so that they can get a reasonable amount of both chemicals. They can then work their way up slowly, based on the THC, from just a few milligrams of THC upward, until their symptoms are alleviated. If, for example, they get up to 10 milligrams of THC, that would mean they are also taking 40 milligrams of CBD, which is a dose that can also help with pain, insomnia, anxiety, and inflammation.

Tinctures come in a variety of ratios of CBD to THC, with ratios as high as 25:1 or even higher. This flexibility is extremely helpful. For example, to alleviate some of the symptoms of autism spectrum disorder—such as anxiety, irritability, and self-injurious behavior—particularly in teens, CBD with just a tiny bit of THC—a 25:1 ratio—is perfect for that purpose. There are also tinctures that contain CBN (cannabinol) to aid sleep, CBG (cannabigerol) to relieve anxiety and muscle pain, and CBDA (cannabidiolic acid), which acts as a strong anti-inflammatory. Some tinctures have other components in them as well, such as melatonin, which is a sleep aid.

Still, you must be cautious about the amount of THC you are consuming, regardless of the ratio. For example, a 25:1 ratio of CBD:THC doesn't sound like a lot of THC, but a gummy with 100 milligrams of CBD—a dose that many people may need—has 4 milligrams of THC, which is enough for some people to become moderately intoxicated.

Tinctures can be based in either alcohol or oil. Generally, oil-based tinctures are preferred. There are DIY recipes and devices for making oil-based tinctures, but for most people it's more convenient to buy tinctures at a cannabis dispensary. On the other hand, alcohol-based tinctures are incredibly easy to make at home. All you need to do is buy some cannabis flower, crumple it up, and bake it in the oven for thirty minutes at 230°F (110°C). Next, put the cannabis in a bottle of very concentrated alcohol (e.g., Everclear) and turn it over once a day to mix the contents. In two weeks, you'll have an effective medicinal tincture. Unfortunately, alcohol-based tinctures tend to burn under the tongue and leave a very strong alcohol taste in the mouth. The alcohol isn't very good for you, so it is usually better to stick to oil-based tinctures, which, fortunately, are typically sold at dispensaries.

## Edibles

For better or worse, you may remember baking and eating lumpy marijuana brownies (parts of which were stronger than others) when you were in college. You may also remember feeling nauseous and overly stoned from eating too much of the infused leftover brownie batter. The science of edibles has come a long way since then. Visiting a dispensary (see chapter 6) can be quite bewildering because of the vast choice of edible products. But buying them can be easy enough, thanks to content labels that list exact amounts of THC and other components in the product.

If you are buying an edible, the most important thing to know about it is the dosage—the amount of THC it contains. Start with a 5-milligram gummy. Do not get upsold to something stronger. If you buy a beverage, make sure it contains 5 milligrams of THC, not 50 or 100, unless you are sure that you need something very strong; but *do not start* with this amount. Be very careful with the dose in a chocolate bar—make sure there are just 5 milligrams of THC *per square*, and not more.

A note of caution: *If you don't know the dose of an edible, do not take it, ever*. Only accept chocolate, a cookie, or a brownie from a friend or relative if you know for sure *exactly* what is in it and also know for certain that the person who made it knew what they were doing. People often accidentally overconsume this way, and it never ends well. Just skip it, unless the edible is wrapped and labeled.

Some good choices for edibles might be as follows:

### *Pills*

This option is not particularly sexy, fun, or yummy. Taking a cannabis pill can feel more like taking a traditional medicine, which makes some people feel more comfortable. With a pill, it is crystal clear what the dosage is, thanks to the label on the bottle, so it is easy to not overconsume. You can be assured of the same dose and effect every time.

### *Gummies and Candy*

When you buy gummies, make sure they are the regular 5 milligram strength, and that the container is labeled with a clear dosage. You don't want to take a 25-milligram gummy by mistake. You can't just ask for a gummy without checking the strength, because they come in varying strengths, some of which will be too strong. If it says 5 milligrams on the package it should be exactly 5 milligrams. Once you have done this, you know that half of a gummy is 2.5 milligrams, or that two gummies are 10 milligrams; then you can easily control the dosage, which is the most important component of cannabis medicine. A piece of cannabis-infused chocolate will work just as well as a gummy, but here are a few things to be careful about:

- **Do not overconsume** just because the edible tastes good. You will regret it an hour or so later, and it could even be dangerous. It can be difficult to stop eating chocolate, especially if some cannabis is already in your system, which tends to make people crave sweets. Measure the dosage carefully. For example, if it is 5 milligrams per square of chocolate and you wish to consume that amount, stop after eating one square, and put the rest of the chocolate bar in a safe place.

- **Safe storage of cannabis products—especially candy—is critical,** so that your four-year-old grandchild or your pet doesn't get into your stash and poison themselves. Edibles need to be treated with more caution than other types of medicine because, unlike most medications, they are tasty. I have heard so many horror stories from people who have inadvertently left three-quarters of an unwrapped, unmarked cannabis chocolate bar lying around, only to discover that someone else has eaten it by mistake. This scenario is always a disaster and can lead to driving while impaired. It is unfortunate and irresponsible of the cannabis industry to produce tasty items, such as chocolates bars, that contain powerful psychoactive medicines. Some of these products contain hundreds, even thousands, of milligrams of THC, which is often a dangerous dose.

### *Seltzers*

Seltzers can be a good option, as you can now buy high-quality seltzers with the dosage clearly written on the bottle. Some seltzers are specially formulated with tiny particles (nanoparticles) of THC, which take effect quickly, often within ten minutes—much faster than regular edibles. Check the dosage carefully, however, as I have seen hundreds of milligrams of THC—far higher than most people are looking for—in some seltzers.

Dispensaries can sell a variety of other products that may seem alluring, too, such as infused honey, hot sauce, ice cream, pizza sauce, and even entire infused pizzas. Even though they can look like fun, these products make it extremely difficult to control the dosage you may consume. How many people can calculate how much pizza sauce they have eaten? It is an invitation to overconsume, and because the labeling on most cannabis-infused food products—"Contains THC"—isn't sufficiently noticeable, those products can also be dangerous for other people in your household. Avoid these products entirely unless you are an extremely seasoned cannabis user and don't mind taking a huge dose. In my humble opinion, we should not be making cannabis into such tasty, difficult-to-monitor food products.

Edibles, in general, have a much slower onset than other forms of medical cannabis. They may be the slowest to act, but they provide the longest relief. Edibles often take between forty-five and ninety minutes to kick in. This can make it more difficult to find the proper dose, initially, because it is more difficult to titrate a medication that has a time delay. You must remember, the next day, how the cannabis made you feel on the previous day, a few hours after consuming it, and to what extent it helped alleviate your symptoms. A daily journal can make this process much easier and more accurate. Simply write down how much you took, when it was consumed, how it affected your symptoms, and whether there were side effects. With this information, you can decide to take the same dose or a slightly higher one the next day.

If a particular dose of an edible doesn't work to fully alleviate symptoms, it is best practice to try a slightly higher dose *the next day* to avoid accidental overconsumption. *Do not double the dose on the same day.* The good news is that edibles provide relief for six to eight hours, so, once you figure out the dose that is effective for you, you can achieve long-lasting relief. Edibles can be a great option for controlling chronic around-the-clock symptoms, such as pain and anxiety. In addition, edibles don't need frequent redosing as often as a person might with smoking. People can often get away with taking edibles just twice a day, a much healthier and more effective option than puffing on a vape pen every few hours. The use of edibles, instead of smoking, also can lead to less tolerance to the effects of cannabis and help preclude the need to slowly increase the dose over time.

Because edibles can take a while to have *any* effect, even after twenty to thirty minutes, many people, especially those who are new to cannabis—and desperate for relief—make the grave mistake of taking a second dose. Then, when both doses are absorbed, they can become way too high, which can provoke extreme anxiety and/or disorientation, and potentially even trigger an anxiety attack. It is particularly imperative to start low and go slow with edibles because, if you take too much, you are stuck with the effects for eight hours. Always adjust your edible dose the next day to avoid taking too much.

Some new edible products, such as seltzers and spritzers, are advertised as "quick-acting edibles," and they often take effect much more quickly than you might expect, due to new drug delivery technologies. It is important to factor that in and always read the label. For example, seltzers kick in a lot faster than traditional edibles—often within ten minutes of consumption. On the other hand, in my experience, many edibles that are labeled as "fast-acting" aren't really that different from regular edibles. Some trial and error might be involved in finding the formulation that works best for you.

## Topicals

Topicals are cannabis-infused creams, gels, oils, or ointments that can be an exceedingly effective way to treat surface-level pain, like a pulled muscle or an irritated joint, when applied to the skin. However, they don't work as well when pain is much deeper than on the surface—a pinched nerve in your spine that is causing sciatica, for example. Under those circumstances, there is no way that a topical could diffuse all the way into your spine. Having said that, virtually any cannabis topical that contains any of the ingredients from the cannabis plant works well. Ideally, I prefer topicals that contain this mix of ingredients:

1. **THC:** In a topical, this is nonintoxicating.
2. **CBD:** A strong anti-inflammatory (pain and inflammation are two sides of the same coin).
3. **CBDA:** The acidic version of CBD, which is an even stronger anti-inflammatory than CBD.

The combination of those three components works particularly well and can be found at many dispensaries. Increasingly, some of the "minor" cannabinoids—such as CBG, CBC, and CBN, which have an anti-inflammatory effect—have become part of the mix in topicals. Topicals can also be used in concert with any of the other cannabis products that have been mentioned, such as edibles and tinctures, and because they aren't psychoactive (i.e., they won't get you high) they can be used during the daytime, before going to work or driving—an added advantage for many patients.

## Suppositories

Cannabis suppositories, either vaginal or rectal, can be quite effective. The idea behind suppositories is to put the medicine where it needs to go. For example, if a woman is suffering from endometriosis, pain from fibroids, menstrual pain, or another type of painful pelvic condition, a vaginal suppository might provide very high local levels of the medication. This can often be achieved with less unwanted intoxication. The idea is to supply better pain control with less of the high. According to one study, vaginal suppositories containing CBD notably reduced menstrual symptoms.[2] Some people use rectal suppositories for painful hemorrhoids or for lower back pain.

One of the obstacles to using suppositories is stigma, and also the fact that some people perceive them to be gross and messy. When suppositories work, however, they work well, and many of my patients prefer them to other methods of consumption. It might be difficult to find either type of suppository (vaginal or rectal) at local dispensaries, but they are slowly becoming more widely available. You can find some straightforward DIY methods of making suppositories from online sources, if they are unavailable locally. They are not particularly difficult to make.

There are many other less common methods for consuming cannabis, such as through nasal sprays, bath bombs, throat sprays, lozenges, and skin patches. What you ultimately decide to use generally comes down to convenience, availability, cost, ease of use, control of dosage, timing of onset and duration, and effectiveness.

### Full-Extract Cannabis Oil and Rick Simpson Oil

Some experts recommend FECO (full-extract cannabis oil) or RSO (Rick Simpson oil), which tend to be highly concentrated alcohol-based extracts from the full cannabis plant. They come in a long, graduated syringe (without the needle), and can be extremely high in either THC or CBD, or both, depending on the chemical composition of the plants they are made from. I've found these gooey, tar-like substances to be both very messy and difficult to dose. The goop can easily get stuck in your teeth and doesn't taste particularly good. It can also get all over the place because of its glue-like composition. You can put the stuff on a cracker to minimize the mess and disguise the taste.

There is some speculation that these oils are particularly beneficial because they comprise the entire cannabis plant, which contains healthful components beyond CBD and THC; and there is an unsubstantiated belief, among some cannabis enthusiasts, especially where RSO is concerned, that very high doses of the oil can cure cancer. There is no scientific evidence, however, that this is true in humans.[3]

## Consumption Methods

| DELIVERY ROUTE | INITIAL EFFECT | DURATION OF EFFECT |
|---|---|---|
| Inhaled (smoking and vaping) | 1–2 minutes | 2–4 hours |
| Tincture under tongue | 20–30 minutes | 4–6 hours |
| Edibles (gummies, brownies, pills, seltzers) | 45–90 minutes | 6–8 hours |
| Topicals (ointments, creams, rubs) | 10–20 minutes | 1–4 hours |
| Suppositories | 15–30 minutes | 2–6 hours |

Now that we've discussed the different component parts of cannabis, and the different ways of consuming it, let's look at why older Americans might be interested in cannabis.

## CHAPTER 3

# Aging Isn't for the Faint of Heart

As we age—or take care of our loved ones who are aging—we eventually confront the reality that aging isn't for the faint of heart. Anyone who has witnessed this process knows that it can be profoundly painful, stressful, frustrating, and lonely. Our society isn't well equipped to serve our aging population. Our social safety net is increasingly in tatters, especially compared with those of other modern, industrialized countries such as Finland, Australia, and Canada. In the United States, there is a vast number of items that Medicare doesn't cover. Many older Americans cannot afford vitally needed services, aides, medicines, or medical equipment. Transportation is often a problem for them, as well, when they are forced to give up their driver's licenses and might not be able to afford cabs or Ubers/Lyfts. To add insult to injury, fighting with health insurance companies and dysfunctional hospital systems can become an unwanted full-time job for older folks in need of vital services. I once heard the problem summed up as follows: Everyone loves their own parents but we, as a society, don't provide comprehensive or compassionate care for our elderly population.

Due to the way our society is organized, many seniors become socially isolated, living alone in homes or condos they increasingly can't manage or afford, and without the resources to adequately provide for themselves. If a senior doesn't have competent, involved children or other relatives who are financially stable and who live nearby, it can quickly become nearly impossible to navigate health, social, and financial demands. This is particularly true of people who live on a fixed income, and who scrimp and save just to pay for the basics. The more poverty is a factor, the more everyday hurdles are magnified.

Challenges compound as our hearing and vision decline, which frequently contributes to social isolation. Many of us slowly become arthritic to the point that the activities of daily living such as cooking, cleaning, shopping, and bathing become increasingly challenging. We experience more pain, diminished mobility, and more side effects from our medications. We develop balance issues, trip, fall, and are at risk of fracturing bones. Our sleep isn't as deep or as consistent, all of which dampens our mood and can affect our memory. Aging, especially with chronic illnesses or chronic pain, can be downright traumatic as people lose friends, hobbies, and independence. Ageism is rampant and many elders do not feel appreciated for the contributions they have made. Many feel invisible and stigmatized.

Our broken medical system can be almost impossible to navigate—even on a good day. Caring, competent primary care doctors are a vanishing species, and most people can't afford to pay thousands per year for a "concierge" doctor. People are forced, due to their financial circumstances, into depressing nursing homes or dilapidated assisted-living facilities. The specter of having to face death, and the pain and suffering that comes with it, is terrifying for most people. Our society provides very few resources—material or emotional—to help people cope with the ultimate life transition.

As we age, we steadily acquire more symptoms, more diagnoses, more prescriptions, and more doctors. Some of my older primary care patients practically have a specialist for each part of their body. The number of medications we are taking tends to increase steadily, too, as new problems and symptoms are diagnosed. Doctors rarely think to discontinue medications. Polypharmacy—being on five or more medications—is expensive and confusing. The more complicated one's medical regimen becomes, the easier it is to make a mistake, miss a pill, or accidentally double a dose.

## HOW CAN CANNABIS HELP?

Symptoms such as chronic pain, anxiety, and insomnia are rampant in our older populations. Cannabis addresses issues such as those through a slightly different mechanism than the usual pharmaceutical approach. With traditional medications, a doctor prescribes a unique medication for each new symptom. If you have pain, you are given acetaminophen, ibuprofen, or gabapentin (and then it's up to you to manage any side effects). If you can't sleep, you are loaded up with trazodone (used as a sedative and an antidepressant) or Ambien. It you are itchy, your doctor will give you antihistamines and prescribe skin lotions. If you are anxious, you might receive a sedative or an antidepressant and, hopefully, a referral to a therapist.

Cannabis, on the other hand, can help alleviate a variety of symptoms at once. It can help your pain, anxiety, and insomnia all at the same time, in a way that can be experienced as pleasant and relaxing. If it is used correctly, cannabis can significantly lower the number of medications that older patients need to take. That is why an increasing number of older patients are using cannabis to find relief from the stress and expense of polypharmacy.

Unfortunately, cannabis can't fix the dysfunctional social systems that tilt the playing field against people who are trying to age with grace and comfort, and it can't prevent ageism, but cannabis *can* help people navigate their symptoms in a variety of ways:

1. It can often help treat a variety of medical symptoms more effectively, and with fewer side effects than conventional pharmaceuticals.

2. It can help cut down on polypharmacy.
3. It can help people continue to enjoy their lives as they age and decline, and augment their ability to transcend ever-increasing physical limitations and discomforts, allowing them to focus on what is meaningful and important.
4. It can help us connect with each other, form communities, and engage in meaningful group activities.
5. It often increases our HRQL (health-related quality of life), an important measure of how we perceive our physical and mental health over time. When you think about it, our HRQL is more important than any other metric of well-being.

How are older patients using medical cannabis? In one study, older patients, among whom pain was the most common symptom, "exhibited a significant preference for oral administration over inhalation of medical cannabis when compared to younger patients, respectively. Among patients taking prescription opioids, most of whom were older patients, 54 percent reported a decrease in use concurrent with medical cannabis."[1]

Many older patients are using gummies to treat their chronic pain, and, in the process, they are taking fewer dangerous pharmaceuticals, such as opioids. I have seen this countless times in clinical practice, and it is a win on all levels.

---

## SALLY

Sally is a sixty-eight-year-old woman who has suffered from chronic joint pain for the last two decades. She has always been slightly overweight and this fact, combined with a strong family history of arthritis, conspired to give her increasingly painful osteoarthritis in the joints of both legs. Over the last five years, Sally endured two knee replacements and a left hip replacement, all done at a hospital in Boston, where she was given excellent care. Every one of her surgeries was technically "successful" but she was left with ongoing chronic pain in her knees and hips that radiated into her lower back. This pain was interfering with her sleep.

For Sally, the pharmaceuticals she was taking to relieve the interrelated symptoms of chronic pain and insomnia were challenging. Tylenol did hardly anything to alleviate her symptoms. Her kidney function was worsening yearly with every ibuprofen and naproxen that she took—and that entire class of medication was no longer sanctioned by her doctor. Sally didn't want to be on opioids at her age because, when she had taken them postsurgically, they caused constipation, itchiness, confusion, and lethargy. On opioids, she also felt that she was at risk of falling, particularly when she got up to go to the bathroom at night. Sally was running out of options.

The most distressing part is that Sally was having trouble sleeping. Few things are worse than lying in pain at night, wondering if you will ever fall asleep. Her doctors had prescribed a variety of sleeping pills, including trazodone and zolpidem (Ambien), but because the pills didn't relieve her pain, Sally kept waking and couldn't get a restful night's sleep. The pills also left her feeling groggy and sluggish in the morning.

Enter medical cannabis. Sally was given some gummies by her daughter, who was desperate to help. Sensibly, Sally started on a low-dose THC edible and was able to find the right dose for herself within a matter of days. For the last several years, she has been taking 7.5 milligrams of THC before bed, which would ordinarily be consumed as one and a half of a 5-milligram gummy, but Sally takes one-quarter of a 30-milligram gummy instead, as it is less expensive.

Since she started using cannabis, Sally's sleep has normalized, and the joint pains that had been waking her up in the middle of the night have stopped. Sally doesn't use THC during the day, because she sits on several corporate boards and doesn't want to be impaired in any way. However, just being treated with cannabis for her sleep and pain issues at night has had a spillover effect, and Sally finds that her joint pain is significantly less severe the next day. In fact, she feels more rested and awake—all of which makes her more functional. She no longer takes any unsanctioned nonsteroidals (ibuprofen, naproxen) or acetaminophen and no longer needs pharmaceutical sleep meds. In short, her quality of life has improved.

---

In Sally's case—and this is a common outcome—cannabis treated several symptoms at once: It treated the pain; the perception of pain as something noxious (i.e., some residual pain was still there but it wasn't as unpleasant a sensation as it had been); anticipatory insomnia; and the insomnia itself. Cannabis lessened Sally's joint pain and extended that relief into the next day, in part by improving her sleep, and it decreased her reliance on more dangerous pharmaceuticals. She reports feeling relaxed and mildly euphoric before going to sleep as she gently drifts off each night. With less pain, she is now able to participate in activities that give her joy and meaning, such as going on walks with friends. Those activities, in turn, improve her mood and energy level.

Sally's experience also illustrates another critical point: Physical and mental health are closely related. They are two sides of the same coin. For a person who has pain or insomnia, it is very difficult to be in a good mood. Conversely, if a person is depressed or anxious, they often feel pain more acutely and are less able to ignore it in order to participate in meaningful activities. This creates a negative feedback cycle and worsens their emotional state. If you can break this cycle, you can make progress. For example, I have had primary care patients who were able to reduce their physical pain simply by getting more sleep, which, in turn, improved their mood. Cannabis can help disrupt the feedback cycle of worsening pain, deteriorating sleep, and depressed mood.

Let's see how medical cannabis can and can't help older patients.

## CHAPTER 4

# How Can Cannabis Help?

Since antiquity, we have known that cannabis can help patients with a wide variety of ailments and medical conditions. Now, as cannabis is being re-legalized in the US, we are re-learning the many ways it can alleviate symptoms and improve quality of life, particularly for our elders. Doctors are still getting up to speed on this issue, however. At this point, many of them have had less experience with cannabis than their patients, and their general knowledge base about how to use cannabis is lacking. Patients are exploring the goals of their care, often with an eye to both improving relief from pain and enhancing their lifestyle, and they wonder if cannabis might play a role.

How do we know that cannabis can, in fact, help seniors? One particularly interesting study from Israel, published in the prestigious *European Journal of Internal Medicine* in 2018, titled "Epidemiological Characteristics, Safety and Efficacy of Medical Cannabis in the Elderly," studied patients for quality of life; pain intensity from cancer and other chronic pain syndromes; and adverse events, such as dizziness. After six months of treatment, 93.7 percent of the patients, whose average age was seventy-four, reported a measurable improvement in their condition. Median pain scores dropped from an 8 to a 4 (out of 10). After six months, 18 percent of the patients stopped using opioid analgesics or reduced their dose. That fact alone might explain why the study found that the number of falls was also significantly reduced in this group of older patients. The main side effects of medical cannabis were dizziness and dry mouth. Most patients reported improved quality of life.[1]

Another study examined chronic pain and insomnia in older populations. They followed patients who were sixty-five years and older, and found that after six months of treatment, 58.1 percent of the patients were still using cannabis. Of those patients, 33.6 percent reported adverse events, the most common of which were dizziness (12.1 percent) and sleepiness and fatigue (11.2 percent). Of the respondents, 84.8 percent reported some degree of improvement in their general condition.[2]

Those impressive results are consistent with what cannabis-savvy doctors are seeing with their own patients. The authors of the study caution—and I agree with them—that special care is warranted when treating older adults with cannabis, due to polypharmacy (there can be drug interactions—see chapter 5), nervous system impairment (e.g., confusion or sleepiness), and increased cardiovascular risk. Cannabis can make you lightheaded, especially if you aren't used to it, and the last thing you need to do is fall and fracture bones. Side effects can be minimized, however, by starting cannabis treatment in a slow and judicious manner, with very small dosages at first.

## CONDITIONS THAT CANNABIS CAN HELP WITH

There are many conditions and symptoms that cannabis can potentially relieve. The most common of these are anxiety, insomnia, and chronic pain—especially nerve pain. Cannabis has been demonstrated to be effective in helping people combat chemotherapy-induced nausea and vomiting. It helps stimulate appetite in cancer patients, older patients, and patients with HIV. Cannabis can help relieve gastrointestinal symptoms, such irritable bowel syndrome and colitis, and it has been shown to help alleviate the muscle spasms and bladder irritation experienced by people who have MS. Some studies also suggest that cannabis can help with the symptoms of autism spectrum disorder and various types of dementia. Cannabis can help patients be more comfortable during their end-of-life care. To learn more about the conditions that cannabis helps, read on!

## Chronic Pain

This is the most common symptom that I treat with medical cannabis. Chronic pain eats away at you and can reliably ruin your mood, sleep, and enjoyment of day-to-day activities. Pharmaceuticals, such as opioids, antidepressants, and NSAIDs, which we currently use to treat pain syndromes, can have noxious side effects and are often only partially effective. Cannabis doesn't make every aspect of pain magically disappear, but it might do the following:

1. Dull pain, by directly acting on the transmission of pain signals in your nervous system.
2. Modify the perception of pain, so it isn't perceived as negatively. This might mean that you still feel the pain, but it isn't as noxious or debilitating.
3. Alleviate anticipatory anxiety around pain. Anxiety and pain are two sides of the same coin and worrying about pain can make it much worse. Lowering pain-related anxiety, with cannabis, makes it more tolerable.
4. Help with pain-associated sleep issues, as with my patient Sally (see page 48), whose pain and sleep simultaneously improved with cannabis.
5. Improve your general health-related quality of life, which, at the end of the day, is what we are all seeking.

For chronic pain, I often start patients on an under-the-tongue tincture with a 4:1 ratio of CBD:THC to make sure there is some CBD in the mix (see chapter 7) to boost the effects of the THC. I have them start with the equivalent of 1 milligram of THC and 4 milligrams of CBD (due to the 4:1 ratio). There probably isn't much effect at such a low dose, but some people are very sensitive to the effects of THC. They might try that tiny dose for a few nights, nonetheless, and then—if there was no effect—the dosage could be increased to 2 milligrams of THC and 8 milligrams of CBD. I advise my patients to increase their dosage of THC slowly, and sequentially, by 1 milligram every few nights. Within weeks, patients usually achieve comfortable control of their pain. Alternatively, they may have a side effect that tells us that cannabis might not be the best medicine for them. For example, some people don't like the feeling that cannabis causes, such as the "high" associated with it or any associated dizziness or sleepiness.

Many types of pain can be treated with less than 10 milligrams of THC, but patients occasionally need higher doses. If there is nerve pain, for example (see page 56), I might add some anti-inflammatory cannabinoid CBDA (5–20 milligrams) to the mixture or possibly some CBG (5–25 milligrams). (See chapter 2 for a discussion of these "minor" cannabinoids.)

Although cannabis works for mild to moderate pain, postsurgical pain usually requires opioids. However, by using cannabis, patients can transition more quickly away from opioids after surgery as they start to improve. Cannabis is safer than opioids, so using it is virtually always a net benefit. After undergoing several surgeries, including three that I had recently after getting hit by a car and fracturing my leg, with the use of medical cannabis I was able to stop taking opioids much sooner. Cannabis can also cut down on the use of NSAIDs. One Canadian study on medical cannabis and older patients found that:

> Older patients comprise a growing subset of medical cannabis patients. . . . This patient population exhibits different patterns of use compared to their younger counterparts, preferring high CBD orally ingested formulations, which they use primarily to treat pain-related illnesses/symptoms. Overall, study participants reported that cannabis had a high degree of efficacy in alleviating their illness/symptoms, and many reported a reduction in their use of prescription opioids, alcohol, tobacco, and other substances.[3]

All of this is encouraging, especially the fact that older patients use more CBD, which is generally well tolerated (see chapter 7), and that they tend to use edibles instead of smoking. The patients in the study cited above clearly stated that cannabis was effective and that it helped them lower their use of opioids and other drugs.

### Nerve Pain

Nerve pain, also called "neuropathic pain," is a condition that is difficult to treat. The pharmaceuticals used for nerve pain are not particularly effective and have unwanted side effects. Gabapentin, or its analog, pregabalin (Lyrica), is heavily prescribed for this purpose, but it doesn't seem to work very well for most patients. In fact, it makes patients feel exhausted and brain-fogged. The antidepressant duloxetine is modestly effective for nerve pain. NSAIDs are somewhat helpful and, as discussed, have toxic side effects on the kidneys. Opioids can be prescribed if the pain is bad enough, but most doctors prefer to avoid them. For sciatica, a short course of oral steroids or an injection of steroids might be prescribed. Fortunately, there is good evidence from the 2017 report of the US government's National Academies of Science, Engineering, and Medicine that cannabis is effective for neuropathic pain.[4]

For some types of nerve pain, such as diabetic neuropathy or small fiber neuropathy, topical cannabis preparations are often effective. You can use a topical preparation that contains either CBD or THC (or both). The best topical preparation, if you can find it, includes three different but complementary cannabinoids: THC, CBD, and CBDA (a powerful inflammatory). If the topicals aren't strong enough, you can supplement them with CBD and/or THC by way of tincture or edible.

## Fibromyalgia

Fibromyalgia is a common but poorly understood pain syndrome that affects 2 to 5 percent of the population in the US. Patients who are afflicted with the syndrome experience pain throughout the body, along with fatigue, depression, headaches, and insomnia. There is no cure for fibromyalgia and treatments are oriented toward minimizing symptoms. Many of the mainstream pharmaceuticals in use have unpleasant side effects and are only somewhat effective in contributing to symptom relief. Many fibromyalgia patients use medical cannabis, which can, ideally, help to alleviate several, if not all, of their symptoms at once.

One study, "Safety and Efficacy of Medical Cannabis in Fibromyalgia," concluded that "pain intensity (scale 0–10) reduced from a median of 9.0 at baseline to 5.0, and 81.1 percent [of patients] achieved treatment response." It also noted that "22.2 percent of opioids users at the baseline reduced or ceased the use of these medications at six months follow-up."[5]

Another study found:

> Nearly half of respondents (49.5 percent) reported cannabis use since their fibromyalgia diagnosis. The most common symptoms for which respondents reported using cannabis were pain (98.9 percent); fatigue (96.2 percent); stress, anxiety, or depression (93.9 percent); and insomnia (93.6 percent). Improvement in pain symptoms with cannabis use was reported by 82.0 percent. Most cannabis-using respondents reported that cannabis also improved symptoms of stress, anxiety, and depression and of insomnia.[6]

Those numbers are impressive and explain why cannabis is increasingly considered a top treatment for fibromyalgia in other countries, such as Israel. Doctors in the US have been slower to catch on, but surely they will as more evidence accumulates.

## Anxiety

Wanting relief from anxiety is another common reason patients seek treatment with medical marijuana. They enjoy the gentle euphoria and deep physical relaxation that cannabis often provides. It is unclear, however, whether cannabis actually improves anxiety over time or whether its effects are only temporary. However, from the perspective of patients who suffer from anxiety, any relief from symptoms is an extremely important outcome.

Treating anxiety with cannabis must be done carefully because its effect on anxiety is very dose dependent. At lower doses, cannabis tends to reduce anxiety and at higher doses it can increase it. Treating anxiety with cannabis is the poster child, so to speak, for the advice "start low and go slow." The last thing an inexperienced patient wants to do is to go into a cannabis dispensary and buy a very high-dose gummy or be given a high-dosage edible by a well-intentioned friend, or by one of their children. Taking too much cannabis, especially as a beginner, can cause severe anxiety or even a panic attack.

To treat anxiety, patients often start solely with CBD (see chapter 7). CBD is nonintoxicating and for many people, it is enough, by itself, to take the edge off their anxiety. CBD is commonly taken as a gummy, a pill, or a tincture. I recommend starting with 10–20 milligrams of CBD and going up by 10 milligrams every few days. When starting out, you might take the first dose in the early evening, or before bed, as CBD can make some people sleepy, which is why it is also used for insomnia. It is important to remember that CBD acts just like grapefruit juice by competing for your body's liver enzymes and can affect the levels of other drugs in your body (see chapter 7).

When CBD alone isn't enough to treat a patient's anxiety, adding a small dose of THC can be helpful. THC should be added incrementally and thoughtfully to your regimen, especially if you are using it to treat anxiety. Whether it's an edible or a tincture, you can start with 1 or 2 milligrams of THC and work your way up to an additional milligram every few days, though there isn't great evidence for using high doses of THC to treat anxiety. I recommend consuming an edible or tincture in the early evening or before bed, particularly at the start, so you can get used to the feeling while relaxing at home.

It's also important to practice good self-care when you're being treated for anxiety. Get plenty of exercise, sufficient sleep, and adequate nutrition, all of which will set you up for success. It is generally not a problem to take cannabis along with other medications for anxiety such as SSRIs (selective serotonin reuptake inhibitors) or mood stabilizers (with some notable exceptions, including fluoxetine and valproate). Be careful, though, with sedatives (e.g., gabapentin, Valium, Ambien, clonazepam), because using THC with them can increase how sedated and sleepy you might feel—and it could lead to dizziness and falls, until you get used to it. Certainly, you should not drive while under the influence of any of these medications.

Many people believe that some types ("strains" or "chemovars") of cannabis are better for treating anxiety than others, but there is limited scientific evidence of that. One study showed that "D-limonene selectively attenuated THC-induced anxiogenic effects, suggesting this terpenoid could increase the therapeutic index of THC."[7] Limonene, which is also found in the rinds of citrus fruits such as lemons and oranges, is one of the terpenes (see chapter 2) in aromatic compounds that give cannabis its smell and taste, and that also have medicinal effects. I look forward to more research in this area.

## Depression

Anxiety and depression are linked to similar parts of our brains, so treatment for both conditions overlaps, whether it involves traditional pharmaceuticals, such as SSRIs or mood stabilizers, or CBD and medicinal cannabis. Cannabis causes a gentle euphoria and relaxation. People find that this effect meaningfully alleviates their depressive or dysphoric moods, at least for a time. Cannabis can help "reset" one's thinking and feeling in a more positive, hopeful direction. As with anxiety, it isn't clear whether using cannabis improves or potentially worsens depression over time, or whether it simply alleviates the symptoms. This is also true of other pharmacological treatments of anxiety and depression.

A study from the New York State Medical Marijuana Program evaluated the effects of cannabis on the mental health of older patients. The program wanted to make sure that cannabis wasn't harming mental health. They speculated that alleviating pain is the mechanism by which cannabis helps mood in older patients.

> Our findings rule out that medical cannabis availability had negative effects on mental health for the adult population overall. We also find that medical cannabis availability reduced past-month self-reported poor mental health days by nearly 10 percent—3.37 percentage points—among adults 65 and above. These results suggest medical cannabis access has positive health impacts for older populations, likely through pain relief.[8]

A 2022 real-world study, which was published in the journal *Drugs & Aging*, evaluated the use patterns of almost ten thousand older Canadian medical cannabis patients who used CBD to help alleviate pain:

> Compositions containing only or mostly cannabidiol (CBD) had been used by 84 percent of the study participants. . . . The majority of older adults reported improvements in pain (72 percent), sleep (64 percent), and mood (58 percent), with 35 percent reporting reduced dose of opioids and 20 percent reduced dose of benzodiazepines.[9]

If pain, sleep, and general mood improve with the use of CBD, it is not difficult to understand that symptoms of depression would improve in tandem. Fewer opioids and benzos mean more lives saved because cannabis is safer. Also, those two types of medication are notorious for worsening depression, so substituting cannabis for them should help with mood.

## Tolerance Breaks

One problem some people encounter when using cannabis to improve their mood is that they find themselves using increasing amounts of it and then use it all the time in a bid to recreate the feeling of well-being and gentle euphoria as the THC wears off. This can be particularly true if you are vaping or smoking cannabis, because the beneficial effects come on rapidly, and although the THC enters your brain more quickly than it would with an edible or a tincture, it doesn't last nearly as long.

Getting into the habit of using increasing amounts of cannabis can lead to a binge/withdrawal cycle that is often seen in patients who are addicted to other drugs. They experience tolerance and withdrawal and need ever-increasing dosages. That tends to be true of people who puff on their vape pens all day, and it results in decreasing effect as tolerance builds. It also causes lung irritation. It is important to try to keep doses from slowly rising over time, and to consider the possibility of addiction if your use gets out of control. If your condition progresses, you might need a higher dose over time, which is not considered tolerance. It is important to monitor one's use and seek help if usage is getting out of control.

Some people take tolerance breaks, or "T breaks," so that their tolerance resets, and they can get back to achieving the desired effects using much smaller amounts of cannabis. This is done by abstaining from cannabis for a period of one to two weeks. It can be difficult to get through two weeks without cannabis in the absence of the symptomatic relief that cannabis gives, however. If you are a heavy user, you might also have uncomfortable withdrawal symptoms that might include grumpiness, poor appetite, vivid dreams, and an increase in anxiety. After a tolerance break, your usage can go back to what it was when you first started medical cannabis—before you developed tolerance. It will be healthier for you and also be less of a strain on the pocketbook.

I believe that a modest dose of an edible taken a few times a day is a healthier choice for people who are treating depression and anxiety with cannabis than puffing on a pipe, joint, or vaporizer every few hours. For older patients who are interested in using cannabis to treat depression, it is important to communicate the fact that you are using cannabis to *all* of your physicians, so that they can incorporate that information into their thinking about any other medications you might need, or the meds you might not need any more.

## PTSD (Post-Traumatic Stress Disorder)

Our ECS (endocannabinoid system; see chapter 2) helps control emotional regulation and the processing of traumatic, deeply troubling memories. Given the central role of the ECS in memory, it makes sense that cannabis can help patients with many of their PTSD symptoms. As the writer Michael Pollen wrote in his book *The Botany of Desire* (2001), cannabis can help us to forget, which is a critical brain function. For example, if we remembered all the details we are exposed to, such as the faces of all the people we saw on the bus this morning, our brains would rapidly become overloaded and shut down. Cannabis can be helpful for patients with PTSD, particularly veterans who are haunted by traumatic memories. It can smooth the rough edges of troubling, intrusive memories and be a component of successful treatment.

## GORDON

By all measures, my patient Gordon was dying. He was dying across the board: physically, mentally, emotionally, and spiritually. In his mid-seventies, graying and bespectacled—and yet still an imposing figure—Gordon had severe PTSD from gruesome combat experiences in Vietnam. He suffered from insomnia, and his sleep was fractured by violent, intrusive memories. He would awaken terrified and drenched in sweat. Disabled by crippling anxiety, he spent much of his time in bed or in seclusion behind closed curtains. Gordon was in a long-term, loving marriage with his high school sweetheart, but his other social connections were in tatters. Gordon's moods were all over the place: He felt angry, lonely, hopeless, anxious, and inadequate. Clearly, something needed to be done sooner rather than later.

As his primary care doctor, I suggested that he consider trying an antidepressant, in addition to continuing his psychotherapy at the Veterans Administration Hospital. I started Gordon on an SSRI—which is, really, the best we have to offer, given that few medications have been shown to be particularly beneficial for the dreadful symptoms of severe PTSD—but he derived no benefit. His psychiatrist then tried several other conventional psychiatric medications. Still no luck. By this point, Gordon was having suicidal thoughts, and though he hadn't yet made an actual plan to end his life, time was starting to run out. I had been witnessing and trying to help with Gordon's slow-motion collapse for several years, with growing alarm as well as a feeling of learned helplessness.

To make matters worse, for several years Gordon had been self-treating his PTSD symptoms—which included anxiety and flashbacks—with about six shots of vodka, twice a day. His liver enzymes were steadily rising, meaning his liver was dangerously inflamed. This type of ongoing insult can lead to cirrhosis and liver failure, and even to liver cancer. Out of options, it was time for us to think out of the box.

I wondered on several occasions if cannabis could help Gordon. It has helped many other patients I have treated, young and old. Gordon was complicated, both medically and psychologically. The use of medicinal cannabis is more nuanced in older adults, and although it can be quite useful, it can also negatively affect memory, balance, and cognition. Gordon's psychiatrist, who had been profoundly helpful, if not particularly successful, with his psychiatric meds, didn't have a strong opinion about using cannabis to treat patients, as it was outside of her frame of reference. She cited the conventional psychiatric wisdom—little of which I agree with—that cannabis always makes psychiatric disorders, including depression, anxiety, and PTSD, even worse. She thought it might be too dangerous for Gordon to use it, given his suicidal thoughts.

I have been treating patients with medical cannabis for a quarter of a century, ever since I earned my medical license. I have been a believer in the medicinal benefits of marijuana dating back to the time when, as a child, I saw how it helped my brother Danny during his battle with childhood leukemia. I saw my brother overcome the debilitating nausea of chemotherapy, regain his ability to eat, maintain his weight, and enjoy what little life he had left with the help of marijuana. It enabled him to feel well enough to strum on his Fender Stratocaster and, most importantly to me, to play with his boisterous twin brother.

Like many of his generation, Gordon was not a stranger to cannabis, although he had not used it in recent years. His earlier experiences were positive, without side effects like anxiety or paranoia. By the time I suggested that he give cannabis a try, Gordon was so beaten down and exhausted from battling nightly with his demons that he was willing to try anything.

We went over the details of using cannabis safely, the different formulations, and dosage. I reiterated that he needed to "start low and go slow" so as not to overshoot a comfortable and therapeutic dose. I asked him to journal about his symptoms and experiences, including how much cannabis he took and which kind, so that we could assess and correct course if necessary. Most importantly, another visit was scheduled for two weeks out, so that there would be close follow-up. We started with an old-fashioned under-the-tongue tincture with a mixture of THC and CBD. Such tinctures were commonly sold a century ago, before we made our grand societal mistake of criminalizing cannabis. Gordon derived some benefit from the tincture but, upon further experimentation, he found that smoking it was much more effective for his symptoms. Doctors don't typically recommend smoking anything, but we also need to practice "harm reduction," which means meeting patients where they are. Smoking gave Gordon immediate and lasting relief.

The effect of medical marijuana was drastic. To start, Gordon could now sleep through the night. Rarely was he awakened by nightmares, and when he was, he was able to self-soothe without relying on alcohol. During the daytime he felt a stark diminution of his anxiety symptoms, the constant feeling of needing to be on the alert for threats, whether real or imagined. His mood was better, and more stable. He came out of his shell and started to reconnect with friends and hang out at the veterans center. He resumed fishing, an old hobby, and soon lost his taste for alcohol.

Once Gordon stopped drinking, his liver tests came back to normal, which was a tremendous relief to me, as well as to Gordon and his wife. His color and energy improved. When I saw him for an appointment several months later, he appeared calm and relaxed for the first time. He even smiled a few times. Getting a full night's sleep, and not constantly worrying, can make a tremendous difference.

In terms of dosage, we weren't anywhere near Cheech and Chong territory. He was taking only one puff, two or three times a day, from his portable dry herb vaporizer. This is an extremely modest dose. While I'm not a huge fan of smoking anything, Gordon wasn't reporting any pulmonary symptoms. A dry herb vaporizer is a safer way to inhale cannabis because it heats the flower to a lower temperature than burning it, and there are fewer combustion products (see page 30). In addition to attesting to his improved mood, Gordon also mentioned that the pain from arthritis in his knees and his hips had lessened—and he was taking fewer NSAIDs, which can harm your kidneys, as well as other organs. It is impossible to argue that he wasn't a ringing clinical success.

---

One certainly doesn't need to be a veteran, however, to have PTSD symptoms. Socioeconomically disadvantaged patients who are traumatized by poverty, lack of safe housing, and debt also frequently experience trauma. I see this every day in my inner-city primary care clinic. Trauma is also experienced by immigrants, minorities, and others who experience discrimination, such as members of the LGBTQ+ community, as well as by people who are addicted to drugs or alcohol, and by victims of sex trafficking and sexual assault. As I discussed in chapter 3, the process of getting older in our society, which has such a tattered social support network, can be traumatic for many. People from all walks of life have symptoms of PTSD.

Cannabis can help patients with PTSD deal with insomnia, nightmares, and nocturnal flashbacks. It can also help with anxiety, mood disorders, and the "hyperarousal" that people with PTSD suffer from. It can help blunt the effect of intrusive memories. However, as noted earlier, it is important to keep in mind that high doses of THC can worsen anxiety and other symptoms of PTSD.

Not all of the data suggests that cannabis is helpful for PTSD. Some studies show that cannabis is "associated" with worsening symptoms of PTSD. One could explain those findings by noting that there is a correlation between patients' worsening symptoms and the amount of cannabis they use to address their symptoms. It is incredibly important to "start low and go slow" when starting cannabis therapy for PTSD to make sure that you don't overshoot a helpful level of THC and end up aggravating your symptoms.

One study of PTSD compared a group of patients who used medical cannabis with a group that did not use it. This is what the study found:

> Over the course of one year, the cannabis users reported a greater decrease in PTSD symptom severity over time compared to controls . . . Participants who used cannabis were 2.57 times more likely to no longer meet DSM-5 criteria for PTSD at the end of the study observation period compared to participants who did not use cannabis.[10]

My clinical experiences correspond to the study's conclusion that cannabis can be quite helpful in many patients with PTSD. However, the issue needs to be further researched, given that the data in this field is contradictory, and that we are just beginning to learn which doses and formulations might be most helpful for patients with PTSD.

Go easy with THC at first. CBD is an ideal place to start, although you will likely need some THC if you have significant symptoms. A respectable starting dose for CBD might be 10 milligrams twice a day, with the dose going up by 10-milligram intervals every few days, so that the next dose would be 20 milligrams twice a day. Note that tinctures are more effective than edibles, due to better absorption (see chapter 7). Once the dose of CBD is in the 100–200 milligram range, you can add 1 milligram of THC to the evening/bedtime dose, if you feel the need to make more progress. Then, slowly advance the dose to 1 milligram of THC two to three times a day. If 1 milligram of THC doesn't work, try 2 milligrams. Remember not to drive after using THC. Also, it is important to let your doctors know that you are using CBD, so that they can watch out for potential medication interactions. Your doctors should also be aware of your use of THC so they can make sure that your clinical condition isn't worsening, which can happen with cannabis.

Some cannabis specialists and dispensary employees recommend an "indica" strain (referencing the name of the woodier, broad-leaved *Cannabis indica* plant) over a "sativa" strain (referencing the taller, thin-leaved *Cannabis sativa* plant) to help relieve the symptoms of PTSD. Indica is purportedly more relaxing, calming and healing than sativa (see also pages 33 and 153). An indica could, hypothetically, be more helpful to veterans with PTSD. However, many studies of the actual chemical components of cannabis demonstrate little meaningful difference between indica and sativa. A lot of the hoopla around indica is sheer marketing nonsense. Don't believe the hype! It is perfectly fine to ask the folks at your dispensary for a generally more calming type of cannabis that can help reduce the anxiety and hyperarousal that come with PTSD. However, in all likelihood that product will not be an indica or a sativa in the true botanical sense.

Another study concludes that medical cannabis can be especially helpful to older individuals:

> There are important differences between individuals aged 65+ years and younger individuals receiving cannabis-based medicinal products. Older aged

> individuals experience considerable improvement in health and well-being when prescribed cannabis-based medicinal products.[11]

For some older patients with PTSD, including veterans, cannabis can be game-changing. If it can help improve the health and well-being of our elders with PTSD, we will have gone a long way toward helping to address this epidemic.

## Insomnia

Good sleep is an essential component of one's physical and mental health. Treating insomnia with cannabis can be gratifying for people who use cannabis instead of traditional pharmaceuticals. Cannabis can have fewer side effects than drugs such as zolpidem (Ambien) or zaleplon (Sonata). With cannabis, people tend to get a restful night's sleep without feeling drugged and groggy the next morning, as they might feel after taking a traditional pharmaceutical.

Recently, I treated an older patient who has transitioned from alprazolam (Xanax) to cannabis as a sleep aid. Not even the most reefer-averse doctor, who thinks marijuana is the devil's lettuce, can argue that cannabis is more dangerous than alprazolam, a highly addictive benzodiazepine. Benzodiazepines can cause falls, sedation, and memory loss, and they can contribute to dementia. Even trazodone, a generally benign antidepressant that we commonly prescribe for sleep, isn't great for older patients because it leads to sedation, dry mouth and, occasionally, cardiac problems.

A quick note on Ambien, which is an extremely popular sleep agent: More than ten million prescriptions for Ambien are written every year in the US alone because it is quite effective at inducing and maintaining sleep. For this reason, Ambien is often a go-to medication for doctors. I often prescribe it to patients, as well, although they are usually younger.

However, in many ways, Ambien is a highly dangerous medication, especially as we get older. It can contribute to falls and dementia, and people can go into dissociative, dreamlike states after taking it. In those trances, they have no memory of what they've done—including getting into their car and driving. Studies have shown that people who take Ambien are twice as likely to get into a car accident as those who don't use Ambien. They might even eat their way through the refrigerator and leave food wrappers all over the place. The next morning, they wonder *Who on earth could have done that?* before realizing that they are the guilty party. Ambien is a good example of a mainstream pharmaceutical that is widely prescribed, but it is likely to be more dangerous than cannabis.

In general, all sleep medications, including cannabis, become more dangerous as we age, because our bodies are more vulnerable to the effects, and there are more drug interactions. All sleep medications are more likely to cause confusion, balance issues, and falls in the elderly. Cannabis, on the other hand, can be a better option for the relief of insomnia (see chapter 5) if it is used thoughtfully and mindfully. By adjusting the dose, one can minimize the risks that accompany using cannabis for insomnia.

Insomnia has several components. Many people have trouble falling asleep. This can lead to "anticipatory insomnia," where they worry about not being able to fall asleep the next night, and their insomnia then becomes a self-perpetuating cycle. I have suffered from this type of insomnia for decades. It is not fun. Other people are in too much pain to sleep or are stressed out and ruminate endlessly on the day's problems. Waking up in the middle of the night to go to the bathroom, and then not being able to fall asleep again, is another problem that leaves people lying unhappily awake, counting the minutes until the morning.

How does using cannabis help with insomnia? What does it feel like when you're trying to fall asleep? People report feeling relaxed and slightly euphoric as a deep sense of calm pervades their mind and body. Sometimes, with higher dosages, pretty colors and patterns bloom in front of your closed eyes—a beautiful, relaxing display as you fall asleep. At the same time, your muscles can feel just as relaxed as they might feel after a professional massage. Often, any pain you feel can be relegated to a quiet place in the distance, where it is not as disruptive. Anticipatory insomnia tends to be subsumed by the pleasant feelings one is experiencing.

As with any other sleeping medication, you must be careful if you have taken cannabis and tend to get up in the middle of the night to go to the bathroom. Cannabis can contribute to feelings of wooziness and disorientation when you get up. There is always the risk of tripping and falling. This side effect tends to diminish as your experience with cannabis increases, but it is absolutely something to watch out for. In general, it is best to have good lighting and nothing to trip over when you get up to go to the bathroom. Get up slowly and make sure you find your balance and footing before taking a step.

CBD is often helpful for sleep, as it can make people feel sleepy and relaxed on its own, without THC. CBD can help treat many of the conditions that lead to insomnia, such as anxiety, restlessness, and chronic pain. I recommend starting with 10 milligrams of CBD, preferably in a tincture under the tongue. You can take it thirty minutes before going to bed. Experiment by increasing the dose by 10 milligrams every few nights. If the dose rises into the hundreds of milligrams range, you may wish to add a small dose of

THC. Start with 1 milligram of THC and work your way up slowly from there.

Smoking or vaping cannabis isn't great for insomnia because the effect lasts for only two to four hours. An exception might be if your only problem is falling asleep—and you rarely wake up during the night—in which case smoking or vaping might be an effective option, if not for the health of your lungs. If you tend to wake up in the middle of the night, however, you don't really want to smoke more cannabis, as it can make you feel more awake—but there are longer-acting options that you can take at bedtime, such as tinctures and edibles, that can help you sleep through the night.

It is usually even better to use a tincture under the tongue for insomnia, because it kicks in within about thirty minutes and can last about six hours. A tincture can keep you asleep all night. Or you might consider the use of an edible, which takes about an hour to act, and can last for six to eight hours—just be sure to consume the edible about an hour or so before you intend to fall asleep. Alternatively, as mentioned previously, you can put a few drops of tincture into a beverage, such as a relaxing herb tea, but it will take as much time as an edible—an hour or so—to work.

It is critical to watch the dose when you are using cannabis for sleep. Taking too high a dose of THC (but not CBD) can be extremely stimulating and make it more difficult to fall asleep. In my experience, this happens, in part, because you can find yourself pleasantly high, and it becomes more fun to stay awake. Then the tendency is to get involved with activities that you enjoy, at the expense of sleep. This is called "revenge insomnia" and, I've found, cannabis can bring it on. Unfortunately, you can also find yourself grazing through the snack drawer or fridge when this happens.

It is critical to practice good "sleep hygiene" to maximize your chances of success with using cannabis as a sleep aid—or with using any other sleep medication, for that matter. Limit yourself to one cup of caffeinated coffee per day and cease all intake of caffeine after noon. Be sure to get daily exercise and engage only in relaxing activities before bed. Studies show that people should not use a bright screen, such as a computer or television screen, for an hour or two before bed. The brightness tells your brain that it is time to be wakeful, not sleepy. Men with BPH (benign prostatic hyperplasia) need to treat this condition effectively because the frequent need to get up to urinate is disruptive to sleep. It can also be helpful to drink fewer fluids in the hours before bedtime.

### RLS (Restless Legs Syndrome)

RLS is characterized by an uncontrollable urge to move your legs, especially when sleeping. Moving your legs may feel like it provides temporary relief, but they can be very sore the next day. RLS can interfere with your quality of sleep and leave you feeling exhausted. It can be extremely difficult to treat RLS, and traditional pharmaceuticals, such as Mirapex (pramipexole) and Requip (ropinirole), are inconsistently effective. RLS can co-occur with both insomnia and obstructive sleep apnea, which is a disorder characterized by pauses in breathing during sleep, inefficient sleep, and daytime sleepiness.

---

### SOPHIE

Sophie was in her late fifties. She was healthy and fit and didn't take any medications or have any medical problems. She developed RLS, which started to interfere with her sleep and made her legs feel sore the next day. Sophie is a very athletic, active person, and the lack of sleep and her sore legs were undercutting her lifestyle and sense of well-being. Sophie tried several pharmaceuticals, including the commonly prescribed pramipexole (Mirapex), to treat RLS, but they made her feel groggy and gave her a dry mouth, among other side effects—not the relief she was looking for. Sophie asked me about treating her condition with medical cannabis, and the results were far better than expected.

With the introduction of a modest dose of cannabis medicine, all of Sophie's RLS symptoms were entirely resolved within a week. We used a tincture formulation that had equal parts THC and CBD. Having used cannabis before, she was able to start with at a slightly higher dose than I would prescribe for a newcomer to cannabis. She started with 3 milligrams of THC under her tongue thirty minutes before bed. The dose went up by a milligram every few nights. By the time Sophie got to 5 milligrams, the RLS was gone.

At one point, Sophie needed to travel and was unable to take her cannabis medicine with her because she was flying to a state where cannabis isn't legal. She was concerned that symptoms would return if she was unable to take her medicine. Even though Sophie was away for two weeks, the RLS symptoms didn't come back. She was curious about that and decided to see what would happen if she stopped taking the tincture. What happened? Nothing. For about four months, Sophie's RLS symptoms were totally resolved, even though she was abstaining from all cannabis products and wasn't taking any pharmaceutical treatments for RLS.

I reviewed the relatively sparse literature on this subject. In 2017, the journal *Sleep Medicine* published a case study of six patients who had RLS and a similar miraculous-seeming response to cannabis. According to this study, "All patients spontaneously reported cannabis use and total relief of RLS symptoms as well as complete improvement of sleep quality after occasional and recreational marijuana smoking (patients 1–5) or sublingual administration of cannabidiol (patient 6)."[12]

After about six months off cannabis, Sophie found that her symptoms were starting to come back. She is currently controlling her symptoms with a very modest use of tincture—just a few milligrams a night—whenever symptoms return. Sophie doesn't feel hung over at all in the morning, and the quality of her sleep has been excellent. This case brings up another important point: Medical cannabis patients must be extremely careful about traveling to, or through, an area where medical cannabis is not legal (see chapter 6). You do not want to get arrested. In fact, there were 200,000 arrests for cannabis possession in the United States in 2023.

---

## MS (Multiple Sclerosis)

About 40 percent of people with MS use some type of cannabinoid, such as cannabis or CBD.[13] They tend to use it for pain, spasticity—an uncomfortable muscle tightness and resistance to movement—and bladder irritability, as well as for insomnia. Traditional pharmaceuticals are often unhelpful, but for many people cannabis alleviates their symptoms more effectively.

There is a good amount of data on the effectiveness of cannabis to treat spasticity in MS patients who use nabiximols (Sativex),[14] a natural cannabis extract that is approved in twenty-nine different countries, some of which are in Europe, as well as in Canada and New Zealand. Sativex is not approved in the US yet, despite conclusive evidence of its efficacy. It is used to treat moderate to severe spasticity in MS and comprises a 1:1 ratio of THC and CBD that is sprayed into the mouth. That dosage is analogous to a 1:1 CBD:THC tincture that I often recommend that is available in most parts of the United States where medical cannabis is legal.

Cannabinoids improve pain and troubling bladder symptoms that frequently accompany MS. The use of cannabis can result in reduced nocturia (getting up at night to urinate), fewer voids, and lessened incontinence. In one study, researchers found that cannabis "has an appreciable effect on ameliorating subjective perception of urinary disturbances and appears to have a positive effect on objective urodynamic parameters, particularly in patients with hyperactive bladder."[15]

Medical marijuana can make a huge difference in a patient's quality of life. MS patients can start with a 1:1 CBD:THC tincture—which happens to be the same ratio present in Sativex—and slowly titrate upward. I suggest that my patients keep a record of their dose, energy, pain, spasticity, sleep, and any bladder symptoms, as well of as any side effects. They should discuss their use of cannabis with all of their health care providers to avoid any risk of drug/cannabis incompatibility.

### PD (Parkinson's Disease) and HD (Huntington's Disease)

According to a recent survey from the Michael J. Fox Foundation, up to 70 percent of patients with Parkinson's disease use cannabis,[16] although other surveys have shown somewhat lower numbers. People are using it to relieve pain, tremors, and anxiety, as well as to improve sleep and quality of life. In another study of patients with PD, it was shown that cannabis can help alleviate insomnia—and without introducing significant side effects.[17]

Yet another study of patients with PD demonstrated that cannabis could be used safely to relieve symptoms. The subjects of the study were sixty-nine years old, on average, and used a "median cannabis dose for PD of 20 g/month with a 10/4 THC/CBD percent ratio." This comes out to less than two joints per day, using more THC than CBD. According to this study, "Over the 1–3 years of follow-up, the medical cannabis treatment regimens appeared to be safe. Medical cannabis did not exacerbate neuropsychiatric symptoms and had no detrimental effects on disease progression." The patients did not need to increase their dose of cannabis. The researchers concluded that "it is not considered a replacement for traditional PD meds, but as an adjunct therapy for symptoms."[18]

There is also some evidence that cannabis can be helpful for the symptoms of Huntington's disease:

> There was strong evidence for significant improvement in the neurologic symptoms of spasms, tremors, spasticity, chorea [involuntary movements of the arm and face muscles], and quality of sleep following treatment with medical marijuana. Analysis of specific motor symptoms revealed significant improvement after treatment in tremors and rigidity. Furthermore, all pretreatment and post-treatment measures indicated a significant increase in average number of hours slept.[19]

This study, and others like it, highlight the fact that neurologists need to become more fluent and comfortable with the use of medical cannabis.

## Cancer and Chemotherapy

Cannabis helps with chemotherapy-induced nausea and vomiting, often more effectively than other medications. Those benefits have been extensively documented in numerous studies, as well as in the 2017 report on cannabis from the US government's National Academies of Sciences, Engineering, and Medicine.[20] Few people would contest that cannabis plays a useful role in helping to alleviate this condition.

CINV is one of the few scenarios where I believe inhaled cannabis might be more advantageous than other methods of consumption. When one is undergoing chemotherapy, the urge to vomit can come on very, very quickly. If one were to consume a tincture, it would take twenty to thirty minutes to kick in, or if one were to eat a gummy, it would take forty-five to ninety minutes for it to take effect, which would likely be too late to keep one from vomiting. When nauseous, the last thing one wants to do is swallow or eat something.

Patients find inhaled cannabis helpful because it works instantaneously to alleviate symptoms. Whenever they feel an episode of vomiting coming on, they can take a puff or two. This does not necessarily mean smoking (see chapter 2). Instead, patients can take a puff from their dry herb vaporizer or a discreet puff or two from their vape pen—either of which is, in all likelihood, a less unhealthy way to inhale smoke. Whether done by smoking or using a vaporizer, inhalation makes it easier to titrate your dose, and because inhalation acts within seconds, you get immediate feedback if you need more medicine. You can also control the size of the puff, the number of puffs, and how long you hold each puff in your lungs.

Gummies and tinctures also have a role to play in CINV. They can provide long-acting relief, which can then be supplemented, as needed, with inhaled cannabis—all of which can dial down some of the baseline nausea, with a longer-acting effect. For this to work, however, you must consume them at a time when you won't throw them up.

The amount of THC that people need for CINV to be effective is highly variable. The process of finding the right dose involves trial and error, careful journaling of dose and symptoms, and a slow increase in dose. Cannabis can also help treat some of the other side effects of chemotherapy. For example, some of my patients have successfully used both edibles and topicals, such as a cannabis cream, to treat nerve pain in their hands and feet. Cannabis can also help with stimulating appetite and reducing weight loss, as well as with alleviating pain and insomnia.

A 2024 study, "Cannabis Perceptions and Patterns of Use Among Older Adult Cancer Survivors," evaluated older cancer survivors in states that don't have a legal cannabis marketplace and revealed:

> Half (46 percent) [of the participants] had ever used cannabis. . . . Only 8 percent had discussed cannabis with their provider [and] the most common reason [for use] was for pain (44 percent), followed by insomnia (43 percent), with smoking being the most common (40 percent) mode of use. Few (<3 percent) reported that cannabis had worsened any of their symptoms.[21]

This study serves as a reminder that many Americans still live in states that do not offer legal cannabis. That is a policy failure. It is essential to know exactly what the laws are in your state, and the best way to abide by them—without sacrificing relief of your cancer or CINV symptoms. With the criminalization of cannabis, desperate and suffering people are put in a situation where they have to choose to either abide by the law or treat their symptoms. It is dangerous that only 8 percent of the patients in the study had discussed using cannabis with their providers. That low number might be related either to their reluctance to discuss using cannabis because of its illegality—and not wanting to get in trouble—or, simply, to shyness about discussing cannabis with their doctor.

## Cannabis and Cancer

Having cancer is a terrifying, traumatic experience that can result in many symptoms, including anxiety, insomnia, acute and chronic pain, and depression—all of which might be alleviated by cannabis. But first it is important to clear up some confusion: *Cannabis has not been proven to cure cancer in humans*. If you have cancer, please work with an oncologist to come up with an effective treatment plan. It is best not to follow the advice of anyone who says that strong cannabis formulations like RSO or FECO (see chapter 2) will make your cancer go away. People can get confused about the effectiveness of cannabis for treating cancer because some animal studies have shown ample evidence that various components of cannabis are highly toxic to cancer cells. I would not be surprised if we used different components of cannabis, as adjuncts to chemotherapy regimens, at some point in the future. Presently, there is no evidence that cannabis can treat cancer in humans.

As for *symptoms* of cancer, however, there is excellent evidence that cannabis can help with pain, the perception of pain, and problems with appetite, anxiety, insomnia, and quality of life. It can also help prevent weight loss. The dosages of THC you need to treat those conditions might need to be somewhat higher for non-cancer-related symptoms. Sometimes, cannabis needs to be taken along with other medications for pain, anxiety, nausea, etc., to completely control symptoms, so it is crucial to discuss your use of cannabis with your oncologist to avoid adverse medication interactions.

### IBS (Irritable Bowel Syndrome)

IBS is a common syndrome that afflicts tens of millions of Americans. The main symptoms include abdominal pain, cramping, gassiness, and alternating bouts of diarrhea or constipation. These symptoms are uncomfortable, inconvenient, and distressing. Cannabis is commonly used to alleviate symptoms of IBS. Unfortunately, few scientific studies on the effectiveness of this practice have been conducted, so we are largely relying on an impressive collection of patient testimonials, known as "anecdotal evidence."

Some experts speculate that IBS, as a disease, might have to do with "endocannabinoid deficiency,"[22] a theory that low levels of naturally circulating endocannabinoids in the body contribute to diseases such as IBS, fibromyalgia, and migraine. This theory has not yet been proven. Regarding IBS, it is thought that the use of cannabis can help regulate the gut's endocannabinoid tone, via the body's ECS (endocannabinoid system), which is why people find it so effective. Indeed, one interesting study concluded that "cannabis use may decrease inpatient health care utilization in IBS patients. These effects could possibly be through the effect of cannabis on the endocannabinoid system."[23]

The cannabis users in that study had a shorter length of stay in the hospital, which made them less susceptible to the many unfortunate things that can happen in the hospital, like medical errors or infection with superbugs.

Although some people can get short-lived and immediate relief from inhaling cannabis for IBS symptoms, I think it is more effective to take an edible or a tincture, so that the various cannabis components can become concentrated in the gastrointestinal tract. A rectal suppository should work as well, but is less convenient, and many patients prefer to avoid this messy option. As with all conditions, determining the proper dose and delivery method involves some trial and error. I suggest working your way up on the CBD, and then judiciously adding some THC, until you feel some comfort.

## IBD (Inflammatory Bowel Disease): Crohn's Disease and Ulcerative Colitis

IBD is a group of incredibly distressing inflammatory, erosive gastrointestinal conditions in the digestive tract that cause pain, bloating, and rectal bleeding. IBD is divided into two types: Crohn's disease and ulcerative colitis. Crohn's can present anywhere in the GI (gastrointestinal) tract, and ulcerative colitis tends to concentrate in the colon. Both are miserable conditions and are difficult to treat. It is estimated that up to 15 percent of IBD patients use cannabis to find relief.

Good data suggests that cannabis provides symptomatic relief, even if it is not entirely clear how cannabis accomplishes this. Cannabis can drastically improve symptoms ratings scores and lower the use of other medications, such as steroids or immunosuppressants, that are also used to relieve symptoms. However, cannabis doesn't appear to lessen the disordered and inflamed cell structures that are characteristic of these diseases. For that reason, cannabis is not a "disease-modifying agent" in the way that immunosuppressants and steroids are.

One study from the *American Journal of Gastroenterology* speculates on how cannabis might alleviate symptoms: "Cannabis binds to the cannabinoid receptors in the enteric nervous system to exert its anti-inflammatory effects leading to symptomatic relief." The study also showed that

> UC [ulcerative colitis] patients without cannabis use appeared to have higher intestinal surgeries and malnutrition compared to cannabis users. IBD with cannabis use demonstrated a shorter length of hospital stay compared to non-users, (4.8 days vs 5.4). They also demonstrated less steroid use (6.6 percent vs 8.2 percent) and

> decreased mortality (0.43 percent vs 1.95 percent). The rate of intestinal obstruction and anemia was lower in cannabis users.[24]

Other complications, such as the development of fistulas and abscesses, were increased in IBD patients who used cannabis, which is of concern. On the whole though, this is an encouraging study of cannabis and IBD.

Another study, out of Israel, in this case using more CBD than THC, echoed the idea that cannabis can help with symptoms, but not with the underlying diseased cells: "Eight weeks of CBD-rich cannabis treatment induced significant clinical and QOL [quality of life] improvement without significant changes in inflammatory parameters or endoscopic scores."[25]

In that study, a CBD:THC ratio of 4:1 was used, which is what I have recommended for many of the conditions discussed in this book, including IBD. The participants used an oil, i.e., a tincture, that they put under their tongues and rolled around in their mouths until it was absorbed. The starting dose was 8 milligrams of CBD and 2 milligrams of THC, which is about the same amount that my patients use to start out. If patients needed higher dosages to quell their symptoms they were allowed to titrate up. The patients ended up using a median dose of 80 milligrams of CBD and 20 milligrams of THC, which is a high enough dose to make most people quite high, dizzy, or sleepy. For instance, I would be pretty stoned if I took 20 milligrams of THC, even with the use of CBD—which can mitigate some of the effects of THC. The key is to get up to that level gradually, if you need it, so that you don't overshoot, can adjust, and will still be relatively functional. In any case, you should not drive on this dose.

It would be more helpful if cannabis could play a greater role in modifying the root causes of inflammatory diseases. As we learn more about the endocannabinoid system, perhaps we will be able to develop agents that can do this. However, at the end of the day, if the health-related quality of life for patients who suffer from these miserable diseases could go up with cannabis, it would be a big win.

If you have ulcerative colitis, most of the pain and inflammation is situated at the very end of the colon, near your rear end, which might be a good indication that you should try a cannabis rectal suppository. The idea is to "put it where it needs to go," giving you better symptom control, with less psychoactive effect, so that you can be more functional. These days, suppositories can be found with more regularity (no pun intended) at dispensaries—and there are many DIY recipes online, so you can also make your own using high-quality, if not sterile, ingredients.

## GERD (Gastroesophageal Reflux Disease)

Some people report that GERD symptoms lessen when they start using medical cannabis for other conditions. One study points out that the gut has a vast number of cannabinoid receptors that secrete less acid in response to cannabinoids, and that would likely help with GERD symptoms.[26] I suspect there's an alternative explanation. Because cannabis does a good job of controlling pain and inflammation, some patients who suffer from GERD often diminish their consumption of NSAIDs—such as ibuprofen (Advil, Motrin), naproxen (Aleve), and others—to relieve their symptoms. NSAIDs are known to be a major culprit in the progression of GERD, so taking fewer of these irritating medicines results in less irritation of the gastrointestinal tract. There is also some speculation that cannabis can help with bloating brought on by gastroparesis, a condition that is characterized by slow stomach emptying and that can also contribute to GERD.

I don't treat GERD with cannabis because there are some excellent, easily accessible, over-the-counter meds for it, such as famotidine (Pepcid) and omeprazole, neither of which has any psychoactive effect, and both of which are generally safe.

## Arthritis

Arthritis is one of the most common indications for the use of medical cannabis products, particularly in older patients. As we get older, and often portlier, our backs, hips, spines, and knees can develop osteoarthritis, or "wear-and-tear arthritis." Cannabis can be extremely helpful for this kind of pain. In addition to edibles—which may contain both CBD and THC, or a tincture with, for example, a 4:1 ratio of CBD:THC—people can also find great relief with a preparation. Ideally, it should contain all three helpful ingredients: THC, CBD, and CBDA (a powerful anti-inflammatory), although topicals that contain just THC or CBD are quite effective as well. A combination of an edible and some cream rubbed into an achy joint can work wonders for hours at a time.

Other types of arthritis are more complex to treat. For example, rheumatoid arthritis is a systemic disorder of the immune/inflammatory system. It is thought that cannabinoids can help tone down inflammation as well as help alleviate pain. According to one study that used Sativex spray (see pages 24 and 76), which is not yet approved in the US, "the large majority of adverse effects were mild to moderate . . . in comparison with placebo." The study goes on to say that "the cannabis-based medicine produced statistically significant improvements in pain in movement, pain at rest, and quality of sleep. . . . No one in the treatment group withdrew from treatment due to adverse effects."[27]

Cannabis is also commonly used for lower back pain arising from muscle strain. To relieve symptoms, you can use a combination of topicals, skin patches, and edibles/tinctures.

## Epilepsy

CBD has been shown to be effective in preventing epileptic seizures in the context of difficult-to-treat childhood epilepsy syndromes. Epidiolex is an FDA-approved medication for this condition. I suspect that CBD will eventually be used more in seizure control regimens for adults, but its efficacy hasn't been definitively proven in this group, although studies are ongoing.

Epilepsy regimens for older adults can be profoundly complicated—and no one can afford to get it wrong, as seizures can be lethal. All epileptic care should be done in close concert with a mainstream neurologist. If CBD, or any THC, is to be added to your treatment for epilepsy, it is best practice to do it along with your neurologist. Do not stop or alter your current antiepileptic medications without medical consultation. CBD can also interfere with levels of other antiepileptic medications you may be taking, by affecting liver enzymes. CBD usually raises the level of other medications in the blood, because it competes with the liver enzymes that break them down (see chapter 7). That scenario can lead to side effects and toxicity—another reason for caution and close monitoring by your doctor.

## Low Appetite and Weight Loss

One of the stereotypes about cannabis is that it makes you hungry and gives you the munchies. I can attest that this is true. After you use cannabis, everything tastes significantly better, to the extent that you can easily overeat. This side effect is not good if you are trying to lose weight. However, it can be extremely helpful for people with diminished appetite or unwanted weight loss, regardless of the cause (HIV/AIDS, chemotherapy, cancer, gastroparesis, chronic pain, old age, etc.)

As people get older, their teeth can give them trouble, and they can also have difficulty swallowing. Our sense of smell and taste can diminish as we age, too, which can lower appetite, and some medications might also have an impact on hunger. Any number of diseases can wipe out your appetite, but it can also just dwindle with age, without any obvious cause. This condition is known as "anorexia of aging." Luckily, cannabis can help get people back on track to maintain their weight and avert hunger by making food more palatable. One study showed that:

> Regarding delta-9-tetrahydrocannabinol (THC), a weight increase of ≥10 percent was observed in 17.6 percent of patients with doses of 5 mg or 10 mg capsules daily, without significant side effects. Additionally, patients treated with THC 2.5 mg reported improved chemosensory perception and increased appetite before meals compared to placebo. No significant side effects were reported in older adults taking cannabinoids.[28]

This study also notes that "Anorexia of aging (AoA) is a highly prevalent syndrome among older adults. . . . AoA links to adverse outcomes, such as alterations in functional autonomy [i.e., the ability to be independent], mood, and cognition."

Therefore, it is critical to stay on top of this condition, if indeed you are suffering from it, and to be aware that cannabis, especially the THC component, has tremendous potential to help. I suggest starting with a 1:1 CBD:THC tincture. This is relatively more THC than I would usually suggest, but you can then slowly work your way up, starting with 2 milligrams of THC, and then go up a milligram each day until your appetite has improved. I also suggest that you work with your doctor and perhaps a nutritionist to see if a medical workup is needed (for example to assess whether there are any problems with swallowing or if nutritional shakes might be helpful).

## END-OF-LIFE PALLIATIVE CARE

When my dad was getting close to the end of his storied ninety-two-year-old life, and as his three cancers continued to close in, he started experiencing worsening pain, anxiety, and insomnia. Medical cannabis was a gift to him. He would use it nightly to alleviate many of his symptoms, such as pain, nausea, and malaise, all at once. Cannabis was the only thing that helped relieve the hot flashes that came from the testosterone-blocking treatment he was taking for prostate cancer. It helped to maintain his weight and prevent him from getting bored and lonely from the loss of all the activities he previously enjoyed. It helped him sleep.

My dad would routinely take a puff or two of cannabis. Smoking would put him into a relaxed and euphoric state. His mood, which had been lowered by the loss of friends, health, and activities, would improve immediately with a puff or two of cannabis. He would smile, and you could see his whole body start to relax. He was more coherent and communicative after a few puffs of cannabis than he was without it. I suspect that was because he had the pain, anxiety, and insomnia under control—without being drugged with pounds of morphine. I was his health care proxy, and I condoned his smoking cannabis. Dad enjoyed smoking and there was no reason to deny him that pleasure at the very end of his life. Why deny loved ones pleasure when their days are numbered?

When the hospice service started coming to his apartment—as the end was in sight—we insisted that he be allowed to continue to use medical cannabis. Hospice workers are wonderfully compassionate and empathic, but their training and instinct is to address most symptoms with opioids and sedatives. Dad's palliative care team wasn't against medical cannabis per se; they just weren't particularly familiar with it.

My dad sensed that he didn't have much time left. He greatly preferred the relative alertness of cannabis to the zombie-like sedation of opioids and benzodiazepines, but as he got closer to the end, as his condition deteriorated, he was forced to use some of those medications as well. We got away with using less of them, however, because they worked well as a complement to the medical cannabis he was using.

Because we used cannabis, instead of the other meds, we were given a gift. The night before he died, Dad was able to participate in a Zoom birthday party (during the pandemic) with all of his kids and grandkids. During the call, he even made a joke! He was so delighted to be participating in such a heartwarming event, which would never have happened if he had been in a sedated trance. Later that night, he passed away peacefully in his sleep, without suffering. It was as if he had been able to say goodbye and knew that it was his time.

---

Cannabis can vastly improve the quality of life for people who are contending with life-threatening diseases or simply dying of old age. For patients with terminal illnesses, a common cluster of symptoms includes insomnia, pain, nausea/lack of appetite, weight loss, frailty, and depression/anxiety. Cannabis can help alleviate many of those symptoms at the same time, and it often improves quality of life. People need to be comfortable and die with dignity. Cannabis, as well as many psychedelic drugs (see chapter 9), can aid that process for many patients.

Using cannabis instead of, or in addition to, the drug cocktails we traditionally use for the dying can reduce toxic side effects, such as profound sedation. One might be able to use lower doses of opioids and benzos to treat pain and anxiety. Cannabis is safe to use when given with opioids and is "opioid-sparing," which means you can get away with using less of the opioid. In fact, they work well together, so there's less constipation, itchiness, and sedation, and fewer falls. Cannabis can also facilitate mindfulness and interpersonal connection, which are gifts at the end of life (see chapter 8). It can help people dissociate from noxious physical symptoms and focus on what is important, such as the people around them. Of course, cannabis does have its own side effects to watch out for (see chapter 5), especially if smoked or given in too high a dose.

When hospice workers come into your life, or your loved one's life, they are 100 percent focused on alleviating symptoms. I recommend that you work with your hospice team to integrate medical cannabis with any other treatments they may provide. Increasingly, hospice teams are familiar and comfortable with blending those treatments. Ideally, doing so can help prevent your family member from being too drugged out in the last hours and days of their lives and, depending on how sick they are, it can help them say goodbye in a meaningful way. Of course, if your family member is in excruciating pain, or is laboring to breathe, morphine is the compassionate option, and your loved one might not particularly wish to still be aware of what is going on.

Amen to not suffering! We can often do a better job with medical cannabis. One study notes that "as this class of therapeutic agents [cannabis-based medicines] are likely to play a major role in palliative medicine in the near future, clinicians would benefit from familiarizing themselves with [them]."[29]

As with so many other areas of medical cannabis use, doctors have a lot of catching up to do.

## Sexual Dysfunction

People tend to shy away from talking about sexuality in older adults, but it is a crucial topic. Many older patients are, in fact, sexually active. Cannabis has been used as an aphrodisiac for thousands of years, and many people report that it substantially improves their sex lives, and for good reason. For one, cannabis indisputably acts as an aphrodisiac, if it is used at the right dosage and in the right setting. There are few cannabis users who would deny this. It vastly intensifies all sensations, particularly touch, and can also help people to mindfully relax into the present. Cannabis has been shown to be helpful with female orgasmic disorder or anorgasmia, as well. According to a study from the *Journal of Sexual Medicine* on post-menopausal women and orgasm, 85 of the 451 women who responded to the survey "stated that they used cannabis specifically to help with orgasm. Overall, 70 percent stated 'It helped them orgasm,' while 24.4 percent stated, 'It helped a little' and 5.6 percent stated, 'It did not help.'"[30]

There is no other drug for female orgasmic disorder.

Cannabis can help couples relate to each other and communicate honestly and meaningfully. The key is to keep the dosage reasonable. If you take an extremely high dose and are profoundly intoxicated, it is unlikely that your sexual performance or enjoyment will be what it could be on a lower, more reasonable dosage. As is often the case with medical cannabis, less is more.

## ASD (Autism Spectrum Disorder)

Most of the studies of cannabis and autism are done on teenagers. Older patients contend with autism as well, and it is likely that many of the results of the studies could apply to them, too. According to a recent study, "The use of medicinal cannabis in treating ASD has shown potential in improving symptoms such as hyperactivity, aggression, self-harm, sleep disturbances, and anxiety. Recent studies highlight that cannabinoids, particularly CBD (cannabidiol), may be a safe and effective option for relieving these symptoms and improving patients' quality of life."[31]

For ASD symptoms, people generally use CBD, mostly because it has been studied for this condition, and health care providers are hesitant to give significant amounts of THC to children and teenagers for fear that it might be harmful. They are less cautious about giving THC to adults. One might use a CBD:THC ratio of 25:1 to ensure that the dose is mostly CBD with a little bit of THC. Data suggesting that cannabinoids might help the "core" symptoms of autism, i.e., challenges with social communication and interaction skills, is limited. The research is ongoing.

## ALS (Amyotrophic Lateral Sclerosis or Lou Gehrig's Disease)

ALS is a brutal neurodegenerative disease that causes progressive weakness and loss of muscle control. Life expectancy for those with this disease is variable. In many states, ALS is a qualifying condition for using medical cannabis. There is some evidence that it can help relieve pain, anxiety, insomnia, depression, appetite loss, and muscle spasms. One study showed that "nabiximols had a positive effect on spasticity symptoms in patients with motor neuron disease and had an acceptable safety and tolerability profile" and added, "No patients dropped out of treatment due to side effects."[32]

Another found that "although research in humans remains limited, a few studies suggest that cannabis and CBD, in humans, provide benefits for both motor symptoms, including rigidity, cramps, and fasciculations, and non-motor symptoms including sleep quality, pain, emotional state, quality of life, and depression."[33] ALS is a devastating disease, and patients who suffer from it need all the support, comfort, and help they can get, including any derived from medical cannabis.

### Alzheimer's Disease and Other Dementias

Cannabis does not cure Alzheimer's disease or any other type of dementia, but it can help relieve some symptoms. My dad had dementia at the end of his life. When he took a puff or two of cannabis, he was more relaxed and comfortable and, as a result, his communication skills improved, at least temporarily. His speech was a lot more fluent and coherent. Cannabis didn't appear to affect his memory one way or another.

For decades, we have been using mediocre medications for dementia, such as donepezil (Aricept), which, at best, modestly slows down the symptom progression of dementia patients. However, some exciting new medications have come out recently, such as lecanemab (Leqembi) and donanemab (Kisunla), which seem to be vastly more effective. Cannabis has not been shown to interfere with the usage of these medications or to worsen memory in dementia patients.

Furthermore, cannabis and/or CBD can improve the experience of dementia for patients by alleviating their anxiety, insomnia, and pain. It can accomplish this in combination with fewer of the toxic, overbearing pharmaceuticals that we readily use, such as painkillers and sedatives. These medications can transiently worsen one's memory. CBD and other cannabinoids have been shown to help with the disruptive and, at times, destructive behavior that dementia brings on and also help with symptoms of other neuropsychiatric conditions that include anxiety, insomnia, and aggressiveness:

> CBM [cannabis-based medicine] formulations containing higher CBD concentrations were associated with improved motor symptoms, such as dyskinesia and chorea, associated with HD [Huntington's disease] and PD [Parkinson's disease]. CBM with higher THC concentration also appeared to show an association with reduced severity of BPSD [behavioral and psychological symptoms of dementia], such as sleep disturbance and agitation. Overall, CBM appeared to be well tolerated. . . . These preliminary conclusions could guide using plant-based . . . cannabinoids as safe, alternative treatments for managing neuropsychiatric symptoms in neurocognitive vulnerable patient populations.[34]

Another study concluded that nabilone (Cesamet), a synthetic drug that is similar in function to THC, "may be an effective treatment for agitation [in Alzheimer's]."[35]

Yet another study reported that "CBD-rich oil is an effective and safe therapy for treating neuropsychiatric symptoms in Alzheimer's patients, while also reducing the caregivers' distress."[36] Caregiver burnout and compassion fatigue are huge issues, and if CBD or cannabis can help reduce them, then the quality of life for both patients and caregivers improves.

CBD and other cannabinoids are thought to be "neuroprotective" in that they can help protect brain cells from insult or injury, as animal studies have shown. Consequently, looking toward the future, it is not impossible to imagine a day when we can prove that the anti-inflammatory effects of CBD and other cannabinoids do, in fact, help prevent the development of neurodegenerative diseases, such as Alzheimer's, Parkinson's, HD, and ALS. Because we lack definitive proof, however, cannabinoids are not currently prescribed to treat those diseases. Their use is best directed at symptom control.

There are many other types of dementia beyond Alzheimer's. For example, vascular dementia is a condition where mini strokes slowly eat away at one's thinking skills and memory. Researchers found that cannabidiol "reduced psychological and behavioral symptoms in patients with vascular dementia."[37]

On the other hand, a recent study titled "Risk of Dementia in Individuals with Emergency Department Visits or Hospitalizations Due to Cannabis" garnered a lot of media attention, because it concluded that "individuals with cannabis use severe enough to require hospital-based care were at increased risk of a new dementia diagnosis compared with those with 'all-cause hospital-based care' or the general population." In other words, those who ended up in the hospital with severe cannabis-related problems were more likely to have a subsequent diagnosis of dementia than those who ended up in the hospital for reasons unrelated to cannabis use.[38]

Although it is possible that cannabis may be neurotoxic in some way, and can cause dementia, as described in that particular study, that notion has not been borne out by many others. I think a more likely explanation is that sicker people have problems with cannabis, and people who have problems with cannabis have worse outcomes. Of note is that people in the ER who were there for alcohol-related emergencies had significantly higher rates of dementia than people who were in the ER for medical problems associated with cannabis. Alcohol, in contrast, is a known neurotoxin, and people in the ER for alcohol-related problems are sicker and on a less healthy trajectory. The "Risk of Dementia" study falls into the category of "hypothesis generating," and further study is needed to make sure that dementia is not a newly discovered harm of cannabis.

## HIV-Related Symptoms

When I was in medical school thirty years ago, a diagnosis of HIV/AIDS was a death sentence. At that time, one wouldn't think of discussing HIV/AIDS in a book geared toward older adults because few, if any, who had the disease would live that long. Now, with appropriate medical care, people are living much longer and doing well. With proper treatment, a patient might have a normal lifespan. Nevertheless, people with HIV/AIDS often suffer from weight loss, poor appetite, chronic pain, nausea, depression, anxiety, insomnia, and fatigue. Those noxious symptoms are often treated with cannabis.

In 1985, the FDA approved dronabinol (Marinol, Syndros), a synthetic version of THC, to help treat appetite and weight loss in HIV. This medication was shown to be effective, which is why it was approved. Patients claim that smoked cannabis, or a cannabis preparation made from the cannabis plant, is more effective than pure THC. It is important to check with your doctor to make sure that the cannabis or CBD you are taking doesn't interact with your HIV—or any other—medications.

## Migraine and Other Headache Syndromes

In 1915, Sir William Osler, known as "the father of modern medicine," and one of the founders of John Hopkins School of Medicine, stated that "cannabis indica is probably the most satisfactory remedy for migraines."[39] I still think that is largely true, despite a century of intensive drug development, but some of the newer medications for migraines seem quite effective as well.

When I was in medical school, I would often come home with crushing, intractable migraines, due to a combination of stress and sleep deprivation from grueling thirty-six-hour shifts. When I got home from one of those endless shifts, and my beeper was finally signed out to someone else, I'd take one or two modest puffs of cannabis to address the crushing pain in my head. It always worked much better than any over-the-counter or prescription medication. Those puffs of cannabis would reverse the nausea and make the pain more manageable. Instead of lying in a dark room, feeling awful until I fell asleep, I was able to participate in meaningful activities, such as going for walks or communicating with friends. I was decidedly more functional.

Generally, I do not advocate for smoking as the safest method of cannabis consumption. However, it can be the most effective method for alleviating an acute migraine. Once a migraine is in full swing, you don't absorb orally consumed medicines very efficiently. That's because a migraine delays the emptying of the stomach, a process known as gastroparesis. If you are trying to get rid of a migraine with pills, such as ibuprofen or Excedrin, it is important to take them as early into the onset of the migraine as possible, before the migraine slows your stomach and inhibits your ability to absorb medications. Many pharmaceutical migraine medications are in the form of injections or nasal sprays to get around this problem. A cannabis tincture, which is absorbed under the tongue, can be effective for migraine relief as well, and it is safer than smoking. An edible is less likely to be effective, as you might not absorb much of it.

Cannabis can help with the pain, the nausea, the anxiety, and the general misery that come from having a migraine. There is no known contraindication to using cannabis along with other migraine medications, such as Excedrin or sumatriptan (Imitrex). Cannabis can help distract you from your symptoms so you can engage in activities instead of just lying there in pain.

## OTHER CONDITIONS THAT CANNABIS MIGHT HELP WITH

There are a number of other conditions that cannabis may help alleviate, including symptoms that range from chronic itching—which is miserable—to painful muscle spasms. It can even help with the boredom, loneliness, and isolation that some people confront as they age.

### Pruritus

Itching can be an overwhelmingly awful and traumatic symptom, if it gets bad enough or if it lasts long enough. It can keep you up at night and drive you crazy. Many dermatological conditions, such as eczema and psoriasis, can cause itching. Metabolic conditions, such as uremia, and certain medications, such as opioids, can cause itching as well. An allergic reaction to a medication can result in profound itchiness—and I have seen patients go out of their minds with itching because of bedbugs. The first step in getting relief from itching is to address the root cause, so that it goes away. You want to make sure that itching isn't simply caused by dry skin, which can easily be solved with the use of a good moisturizer or a humidifier. New drugs, medications, detergents, soaps, foods—or travel, for that matter—might cause allergic reactions or infestations. Pay attention to any other symptoms that might have arisen at the same time, such as fever or rash, and discuss them with your doctor.

## ANNE

Anne was in her early fifties, and in excellent health, when she started to develop angry red bumps on her torso, back, and arms. The bumps continued to spread over several other parts of her body as well, and began to keep her up at night because they were so itchy. Antihistamines such as Allegra, Zyrtec, and Benadryl had little effect. The more Anne scratched, the more the bumps itched, but she couldn't help scratching them. She was going out of her mind. The lack of sleep and constant torture affected her mood. Her anxiety and depression started to skyrocket, and she was snapping at the people she loved.

Anne tried to see her dermatologist, but he was busy and pawned her off on an inexperienced nurse practitioner. Anne was misdiagnosed as having eczema, and was given a moderate-strength steroid cream that didn't do much. She saw the nurse three times, who reiterated the misdiagnosis and slightly increased the strength of the ineffectual creams she'd prescribed. The problem went on for over a year and even turned a highly anticipated family vacation to Europe into a disaster.

Nothing worked to help alleviate the itchiness. The industrial-strength steroid pills Anne was eventually given didn't do anything, either. The only thing that provided relief was smoking cannabis, although I recommended that she use an edible or a tincture instead. Within seconds to minutes of Anne's taking the first puff, the itchiness would get much better. It didn't go away entirely, but it was diminished to the point where Anne could ignore the itching for hours on end. She was even able to get some sleep at night, although it was often intermittent, as smoked cannabis only lasts for several hours. After a while, Anne started taking edibles before bed, which gave her more long-lasting relief.

Finally, tired of this chronic condition, and of needing to rely on cannabis every night for partial symptom control, Anne insisted on seeing her dermatologist. After looking at her skin for two minutes and doing a quick biopsy, he diagnosed her with guttate psoriasis, a super-itchy, inflammatory type of psoriasis. He gave her an effective pharmaceutical regimen for this condition, which cleared it up right away. Now, Anne only uses cannabis when she has a flare-up and is waiting for her traditional meds to beat back the psoriasis.

---

Cannabis is widely reported by patients to help them cope with chronic itching conditions, and various studies confirm this indication.

> Human studies . . . have consistently shown significant reductions [with cannabis use] in both scratching and symptoms in chronic pruritus. Clinical studies have shown a reduction in pruritus in several dermatologic (atopic dermatitis, psoriasis, asteatotic eczema, prurigo nodularis, and allergic contact dermatitis) and systemic (uremic pruritus and cholestatic pruritus) diseases.[40]

## Skin Wrinkles

A tremendous amount of research[41] is going into the production of cosmetics that contain CBD, while the cannabis industry itself is making many unsubstantiated claims about the wonders that CBD can work on skin conditions. Those claims are based on the idea that because CBD is such a potent anti-inflammatory, it can help slow or reduce the formation of wrinkles—and result in healthier skin—when it is applied as a cream. Another claim is that CBD can help with the deterioration of skin as we age. I think the jury is still out on whether any of those claims will be borne out as advertised, since none of them have yet been proven. That fact, however, won't stop the cosmetic industry from marketing product after product that contains CBD for wrinkles and other skin conditions. So—buyer beware!

The beauty industry isn't the only one to tout the anti-inflammatory power of CBD. Pharmaceutical companies, for example, are making similar claims that various creams, oils, salves, and ointments containing CBD can help with inflammatory conditions such as atopic dermatitis and psoriasis. In general, my advice is to wait until there is more data that proves that topical CBD can actually help heal or soothe skin conditions like those. If you are curious, it certainly wouldn't hurt to try various topical CBD products—they are entirely harmless but can be quite expensive. CBD might help with itching and inflammation, but it has yet to be demonstrated that it helps prevent wrinkles, as claimed.

## Muscle Spasms

Cannabis can be extremely effective for the relief of muscle spasms, which is why so many people with conditions like MS use it. It is also helpful for the uncomfortable muscle spasms the rest of us get from time to time—when recovering from a vigorous workout, for example. Cannabis can help alleviate the pain of sore muscles or muscle strains. It doesn't automatically make spasms disappear, but, with the correct dose, it can deeply relax your muscles. If you take the right type and formulation—which may take a little trial and error—you can find yourself in a physically and mentally relaxed state. Your muscles can feel as if they have just been massaged, and the pain can be perceived as a distant sensation.

Pharmaceutical muscle relaxants, such as cyclobenzaprine (Flexeril), tizanidine (Zanaflex), or diazepam (Valium) are effective medications for muscle spasm, as well. The problem is that they make you extremely sleepy and are difficult to take during the day. Even if taken before bed, they can leave you feeling groggy when you wake up. Of course, cannabis can cause a different type of psychoactive effect—you can feel high, which can be just as challenging to deal with during the day, if you need to work or drive. To relieve muscle spasms, you might use mostly CBD or very low doses of THC, and, if needed, add more THC to the dose at night. Hot showers, topical rubs, including cannabis or CBD rubs, and massages are also helpful for tight, spasming muscles.

### Boredom, Loneliness, and Isolation

Many elderly people suffer from boredom as they have more time on their hands. It can worsen, along with symptoms of isolation, as aging people gradually lose spouses, family members, friends, and companions, and as they accumulate physical limitations. Those limitations can also make it more difficult to participate in the pleasurable communal activities that help us to meaningfully pass the time. For example, you might have had to stop playing tennis after a fall or surgery, or perhaps you've had to stop playing music with others because you've developed arthritis in your hands. Alternatively, you may not feel as cognitively sharp and able to participate in challenging games such as bridge or Scrabble as you once were.

As discussed in chapter 3, the later years of our lives can be lonely, isolating times for many of us. This is particularly true of people who aren't surrounded by a nurturing family and who don't have a robust social network or live in an uplifting communal environment. Isolation can deepen when you lose your spouse or are estranged from your kids and grandkids, who might live thousands of miles away. People are often bunkered in their aging houses, which they can't really manage or afford anymore, with too many stairs to contend with and chores to complete. Some elders land in depressing assisted-living facilities or nursing homes.

Obviously, cannabis can't fix the structural flaws in our society that result in so much sadness, loneliness, and dislocation in our elderly population, but there are ways in which it can help alleviate some of the symptoms of isolation and foster connection. If people treat their pain, anxiety, and insomnia with cannabis, and feel better, they will be more apt to reach out and connect with others. Being relatively well-rested and pain free opens the possibility of engaging with others and participating in meaningful shared activities. If your hip pain is under better control, why not swing by the senior center and see what's happening? Why not have a neighbor over for tea? Why not go for a walk or play cards with a friend?

Health is everything, and it is worth putting a tremendous amount of effort into it. You simply can't do as much as you'd like to do if your health does not allow it. This is why, as a primary care doctor, I urge my patients to make their physical well-being the absolute top priority. The healthier you are, the more social activities and groups you can participate in, and the less you will suffer from loneliness.

Cannabis can help us connect with others to the extent that it helps us feel better physically and emotionally. It can quell our anxiety, social or otherwise. It can change our focus from our pain and our misery to the fun we could be having. It can make us feel more rested after a good night's sleep. It can give us the extra boost we need to get out of the house—or out of bed, for that matter. It can help us connect with others. To quote the famous astronomer Carl Sagan, the smartest person I have ever met, from my dad's 1971 book *Marihuana Reconsidered*: "The illegality of cannabis is outrageous, an impediment to full utilization of a drug which helps produce the serenity and insight, sensitivity, and fellowship so desperately needed in this increasingly mad and dangerous world."[42]

Fortunately, that illegality is changing. What better antidote to isolation is there than fellowship? Amen to that! People can form cannabis social clubs or medical cannabis discussion groups and use cannabis together. Those enjoyments are further discussed in chapter 8, which goes into the many ways, beyond pure health and wellness, that cannabis can help with lifestyle improvement.

Some contradictory data suggests that there is an association between cannabis use in older adults and feeling lonely, perhaps because "older adults who use cannabis may experience dizziness and impaired short-term memory, which also prevents them from experiencing meaningful social interactions with others."[43] This study, however, seems to focus almost exclusively on the side effects of using medical cannabis, rather than the benefits of using it. In any event, those particular side effects can often be abated with the use of more CBD (which doesn't cause these side effects) and lower amounts of THC. The study adds that:

> Older adults who are regular cannabis users already manage multiple health conditions (such as chronic pain), making it harder for them to maintain social relationships and social interactions. Among our participants, significantly higher proportions of older adults who used cannabis in the past 30 days were living in a household with two or fewer persons, and having five or fewer close friends and relatives reflect the reality of smaller network size among regular cannabis users. A significant association between a smaller network size and greater loneliness among older adults is supported in this study and others.[44]

A sensible interpretation of this study is that these lonely people are already lonely and are using cannabis to treat their misery. It does not necessarily suggest that these adults are lonely as a side effect of using cannabis. In other words, in all likelihood their use of cannabis is not the cause of their loneliness but, rather, an attempt to alleviate it. However, if you, like some of the patients in the study, are experiencing significant side effects that are not helping you socially, it would be a good idea to reevaluate your use of cannabis. I suspect that, overall, it will help you feel better and connect more meaningfully with others.

A different study on well-being in older adults showed that "older aged individuals experience considerable improvement in health and well-being when prescribed cannabis-based medicinal products."[45]

What about using cannabis by yourself? Is it sad and lonely or can it make you feel happier, more energized, and more engaged? A friend of mine once stated that drinking alcohol alone is depressing, but using cannabis isn't. Based on the totality of what both alcohol and cannabis do for you, I more or less agree with his assessment, although it often depends on the circumstances. Cannabis can help you engage more deeply in hobbies, such as listening to music or reading, but you certainly don't want to spend most of your time being alone, either stoned or drunk—that would be unhealthy. Cannabis is likely most useful when fostering social connections, not just dulling loneliness.

## Potential Improvements in Cognitive Functioning

One theory about how cannabis might help older people to alleviate some of the misery of aging can be gleaned from the work of a brilliant colleague of mine: Dr. Staci Gruber at Harvard Medical

School's McLean Hospital. Dr. Gruber had been studying cannabis users for decades and was curious to know whether medical cannabis users experience the same cognitive effects (e.g., changes or decrements in executive function) as recreational users. Unexpectedly, Dr. Gruber's studies showed that medical patients were found to have improved cognitive function.[46]

Several possible explanations were suggested. The most obvious one is symptom alleviation. People with better mood and sleep, and with better-controlled chronic pain, will be able to think more clearly if they're less exhausted and anxious in general. That's true for most of us after a good night's sleep. Alternatively, maybe is it a question of product choice. Medical users often/ideally select products with lower levels of THC and, increasingly, with different, more healthful cannabinoids, such as CBD and other minor cannabinoids. Age of onset might be an alternative explanation, as most recreational users start in their teens, when the brain is more vulnerable, while many medical users start using cannabis in adulthood. Finally, due to the relief they found with cannabis, medical cannabis users were using fewer other medications, such as opiates and benzodiazepines (e.g., Valium, Ativan), which in themselves can greatly interfere with cognitive functioning. As the authors of one of Dr. Gruber's studies observed, "Patients may think more clearly if they feel better overall."[47]

## Long Covid Symptoms

Long Covid is poorly understood, and it is a clinical nightmare for those who experience it. It is estimated that at least 5 to 8 percent of people who survive Covid end up with long Covid symptoms. Some studies show much higher rates. This translates into at least hundreds of thousands of cases in the US alone. Long Covid is likely underdiagnosed because not everyone knows if or when they were infected with it. I have patients who are anti-vaxxers and who would never get the Covid shot. When they develop symptoms consistent with long Covid, they often don't actually believe that they ever had Covid and reject it as an explanation for their symptoms.

The symptoms of long Covid are highly variable but commonly include fatigue, unstable heart rate, headaches, malaise, weakness, and flu-like symptoms. Long Covid can last for years. There are no traditional medications that have definitively been proven to help treat the symptoms or improve the disease. Long Covid is a new disease, so there just hasn't been much time to conduct research trials on potential treatments. At the moment, we use off-label drugs such as metformin (Glucophage), nicotine (in a patch), or naltrexone—but the data for these treatments isn't at all definitive. Cannabis is thought by many long Covid patients to help with a variety of specific symptoms, such as pain, headache, depression, anxiety, and insomnia.

Cannabis could hypothetically help long Covid patients in ways beyond mere symptom control. Long Covid it is thought to be caused, at least in part, by out-of-control inflammation. Having been triggered by the Covid virus, the body's immune and inflammatory system goes berserk and becomes damagingly hyperactive. Researchers are particularly interested in studying CBD because it is such a powerful anti-inflammatory. There is hypothetical interest in using other anti-inflammatory cannabinoids such as CBD, CBDV, CBDA, CBG, and CBC to help Covid patients, but further study is required. Meanwhile, members of the cannabis industry must refrain from saying "CBD cures Covid or Long Covid," as this has not been demonstrated yet. Such statements mislead patients and give them false hope.

## DANA

Dana, one of my primary care patients, had recovered uneventfully from a moderately severe bout with Covid, but one persisting side effect was the loss of smell and taste. This didn't particularly bother her in the beginning, but by the time she came to my office several months later, she was quite concerned about her weight. As her PCP, I had often encouraged her to lose a few pounds to help stave off future diabetes, heart disease, and arthritis. I was shocked to find that she had lost twenty-five pounds in about six months. This was too much. Her weight was in free fall, she wasn't eating, and we were both quite worried.

According to Dana, food wasn't at all palatable after she lost her sense of smell and taste. She was worried about losing weight and tried to maintain it by focusing on eating fattening foods, but to no avail. She tried nutritional shakes and found that she couldn't force herself to drink them. Eating had become unpleasant, a chore, and it made her feel vaguely nauseous. I recommended that she try medical cannabis, knowing that it can help stimulate the appetite (i.e., it can give people the munchies and make food taste better). Even though she had never tried cannabis before, even in college, she was in desperate enough straits to try it. Cannabis is often helpful with other conditions where weight loss is a problem, such as cancer and HIV/AIDS. There was no reason to think that it might not be helpful in this scenario.

Dana started with a half of a gummy, just 2.5 milligrams. She eventually ended up taking a modest dose of one 5-milligram gummy two or three times a day. Fortunately, she worked from home and this low dose of cannabis wasn't particularly impairing—once she got used to it, after a few weeks—and she could get her work done (although I strongly cautioned against driving). Dana's appetite returned almost immediately when she got up to a 5-milligram dose. She was able to eat and gained back all the weight she had lost including, of course, the few pounds that I had originally wanted her to lose. Slowly, over the next year, her sense of smell and taste came back, and she no longer uses cannabis at all, although she has become a big fan of the idea of medical marijuana.

---

One study helps demonstrate the usefulness of cannabis for treating long Covid. It goes over the evidence, which is not particularly robust, discusses the theoretical rationale of using cannabis for the condition, and concludes that "cannabis-based medicinal products may be effective at reducing symptoms often associated with long Covid, including pain, anxiety, depression, fatigue, sleep, headaches, and cognitive dysfunction."[48]

If that conclusion pans out, it will be a major advance, as we don't have very effective medications for long Covid symptoms—at least not right now.

## CONDITIONS THAT CANNABIS ISN'T KNOWN TO HELP WITH

One thing about cannabis is that there has always been a lot of nonsense about it in the public discourse. This has come both from cannabis advocates, who idealize the plant, and from detractors, who have been indoctrinated by a seventy-year propaganda campaign against cannabis. As we are discussing the medicinal benefits of cannabis, it is also important to be clear about the conditions that cannabis can't alleviate.

- **Cannabis does not cure cancer.** Cannabis can help with the symptoms of both cancer and the chemotherapy used to treat cancer. It has not been shown, in humans, to help fight cancer cells in a clinically meaningful way.

Different components of cannabis, such as CBD and CBG, can kill cancer cells in the test tube, and even in some animal studies, but that is a long way from being demonstrated to be an effective treatment in humans. If you have cancer, work with your oncologist toward a cure, and use cannabis to treat the symptoms.

- **Cannabis does not cure Covid.** Cannabis does not prevent Covid. It has not been shown to help people who have Covid, except perhaps with some symptoms of long Covid. It is recommended that you not smoke or vape anything while you have Covid, as there is no need to further irritate your lungs. It is best to stick to edibles or tinctures, if you are going to use cannabis.
- **Cannabis has not been shown to be a stand-alone treatment for epilepsy in adults.** Some very specific childhood epilepsy syndromes are treated with the FDA-approved medication Epidiolex. If you are an adult with epilepsy and wish to potentially add CBD or cannabis to your regimen, please work with your neurologist. Cannabis may also help with symptoms of antiepileptic medications, if they are bothering you.
- **Cannabis is not a mainstream cure for glaucoma.** There are much better treatments for this condition, including medicinal eye drops. If you have glaucoma, please work with your ophthalmologist and glaucoma expert and do not try to rely on cannabis. Cannabis has been used for glaucoma, and it does lower interocular pressures, but isn't as good as traditional pharmaceuticals for this condition.
- **Cannabis is not a good treatment for asthma.** There are better treatments for asthma. People think that cannabis can help asthma because THC is a bronchodilator, which means that it can open the small airways in your respiratory system. Smoking cannabis

would almost certainly undermine this effect and would do the opposite, by irritating the airways. We have much more effective treatments, such as inhalers, for opening them. If you have asthma, COPD, or emphysema, a good rule of thumb is not to smoke anything. If a cannabis edible helps your asthma, that is a win, but you should still have a conventional inhaler on hand.

- **Cannabis has not been shown to cure or impact the natural course of dementia, Alzheimer's, or any other form of cognitive decline.** Cannabis can help with some of the symptoms of dementia, such as agitation and anxiety, as well as with caregiver burnout, as described on page 95.

CHAPTER 5

# Potential Harms of Cannabis for Older Patients (and Others)

As is the case for all other drugs and medicines, cannabis has numerous harms to watch out for—some of which can be particularly worrisome in an older patient population. To be aware of these harms is to be able to mitigate or perhaps avoid them altogether. Cannabis doesn't work for everyone and not everyone tolerates it. If you suffer from severe side effects, cannabis isn't the right medicine for you.

## ADDICTION

There is no question that, like many other drugs, cannabis can be addictive, particularly because it can bring on feelings of euphoria and a sense of relaxation. In fact, some cannabis users become addicted to the pleasures that cannabis can provide and use it to escape from their daily lives. If someone is addicted to cannabis it generally means that they have lost control of their usage—they are using more and more of it and using it to their detriment. The rate of cannabis addiction is higher in teenagers than adults, although the exact number of people who are addicted to cannabis is subject to debate.

One reason it is difficult to say how many people are addicted is that our official definition of cannabis addiction is broken. Unfortunately, it was created by doctors who didn't have any experience treating patients with medical cannabis, and who didn't seem to understand or even believe in the effectiveness of medical marijuana. That official take on cannabis, which was first conceptualized during the war on drugs—and has never really transcended its political roots—exaggerates how often medical marijuana patients get addicted to cannabis. However, when patients use marijuana medically, at a stable dose, and with good benefit, they are most likely not addicted.

The outdated definition of marijuana addiction or "cannabis use disorder" is that you are addicted if you have tolerance for marijuana (you need more of it over time to get the same effect) and if you are in withdrawal from marijuana (you experience symptoms with abrupt discontinuation of it). That definition of addiction, however, is not used for other medications; there is a double standard for cannabis. For example, people have tolerance for—and experience withdrawal from—many drugs and medications, including opioids (used to relieve pain, primarily), antidepressants, benzodiazepines (used to treat anxiety, insomnia, and seizures), and even coffee—but we don't consider them to be harmfully addicted, based on a definition of addiction that applies only to those who use cannabis. Consequently, medical cannabis patients who are doing well can get saddled with an unhelpful diagnosis of addiction, due to a wrong-headed definition of it, as well as lingering stigma among certain types of doctors.

So, who is addicted to cannabis?

The best definition of drug addiction is "continued use, despite negative consequences." If, for example, you continue to use cannabis, or any other drug for that matter, despite having an adverse reaction to it, you might be considered addicted. For example, if a patient develops CHS (cannabis hyperemesis syndrome, discussed on page 122) and has uncontrolled vomiting when they use cannabis but continues to use it daily, and frequently ends up in the ER and requires IV medications, that suggests an addiction.

Warning signs of a potential cannabis addiction include ever-increasing dosage; escalating, out-of-control usage; and ongoing use despite negative effects on one's life. People who are addicted tend to puff away all day, with diminishing benefit. I dealt with one patient recently who was taking fifty puffs per day on his vape pen. There is no universe in which that level of consumption can be considered medical usage. Another patient asked me for a medical card when he was taking thirty-five puffs a day on his vape pen, and I had to decline his request out of fear that it might only support his addiction.

In medical patients, cannabis addiction is always something to be on the lookout for, in the same way that we monitor the potential for addiction among patients who use opioids or sedatives. If you think that your use of cannabis is accelerating—if you are using it more and more—and are having trouble controlling it, please speak with your physician. One note: If you have a condition, such as osteoarthritis, and it is progressing, you might need a higher dose to alleviate symptoms. In a case like that, using more cannabis is not necessarily considered an addictive behavior.

Cannabis addiction can be quite harmful and has been associated with poorer educational achievement and worsening health. To put it all in context, however, no one has ever died from a cannabis addiction. In fact, cannabis addiction tends to be less destructive and deadly than an addiction to opioids, cocaine, or alcohol. One study observed that "there have been zero overdose deaths attributed to cannabis, and the treatment of cannabis-related psychopathology pales in comparison to both opioid use disorder and opioid related mortality."[1]

In any case, addiction is addiction, and it is important for clinicians to recognize it as early as possible. If someone you love becomes addicted to cannabis, they need to be assessed and treated with empathy, skill, and compassion, just as is true of people with all other addictions.

## CARDIAC PROBLEMS

Data about whether cannabis contributes to cardiac problems, such as arrythmias (irregular heartbeats), myocardial infarction/heart attack (blocked blood flow to part of the heart), and stroke (damage to the brain) is contradictory, but there have been several recent studies that give cause for concern. Most of the studies that suggest risk "associate" cannabis use with negative outcomes. Medical cannabis users tend to be sick already, which is why they use cannabis to alleviate symptoms in the first place. That scenario frequently provides a valid alternative explanation for the association of cannabis use with negative outcomes, making it difficult to ascertain whether any particular harm is directly due to the use of cannabis. Many prior studies have failed to factor in other concerns, such as poverty and the use of drugs and tobacco, that confuse the results. All that said: With cannabis and cardiac issues, I believe that the saying "where there's smoke, there's fire" often applies.

If cannabis can contribute to or trigger cardiac problems, which I believe is the case, it is plausibly due to smoking cannabis, rather than the cannabis itself, for example in the form of gummies and tinctures. When we say that we have studied "cannabis," we have mostly studied smoked cannabis, which is almost certainly more harmful than other methods of cannabis ingestion, due to the combustion products that are produced. Cannabis smoke contains tar, benzene, carbon monoxide, and polycyclic aromatic hydrocarbons, all of which are known to contribute to cardiac disease. We have not studied or concluded that edibles or tinctures cause cardiac problems, because, of course, they don't produce combustion products from cannabis smoke.

Cannabis use hasn't been studied very much in older patients in general, or, for that matter, in older patients with cardiac risk factors or cardiac disease. Another limitation of our database is that we have almost exclusively studied recreational cannabis use and, as we have seen from many studies, medicinal use can have much more healthful effects, due to a variety of cannabis products and dosages. Finally, because cannabis was not legal in most localities—at least not until the last decade or two—we have studied only the effects of illegal cannabis. With its impurities and lack of regulation, illegal cannabis is much more dangerous on all levels, which could skew the data set toward finding harms.

We'll do our best to navigate this field of incomplete data.

Cannabis, particularly smoked cannabis, can increase your heart rate and blood pressure, especially if you take a dose that's too high. It can also cause acute anxiety. Anything that increases heart rate, or that can cause anxiety, will increase one's sympathetic tone (our fight-or-flight response). This could trigger arrythmias, such as atrial fibrillation. Too high a dose of cannabis can place a lot of additional stress on the heart. This is particularly true of inexperienced users, who don't know the proper dose and aren't used to the effects. They are likely to feel more anxiety. Some speculate that smoking cannabis can induce a transient pro-inflammatory state that can make people even more vulnerable to heart attacks.

On the other hand, poorly treated pain, insomnia, and anxiety can also raise blood pressure and heart rate and thus increase one's risk of cardiac problems. Other medications that one might use instead of cannabis can also cause heart problems. For example, NSAIDs, which millions of people use for chronic pain instead of cannabis, cause about ten thousand heart attacks in the US every year.[2] We don't know which is worse: to use cannabis or taking drugs that are harmful, or to leave serious health conditions untreated. The latter, of course, would be inhumane. Cannabis users have been shown to use fewer drugs, such as NSAIDs, that are dangerous to the heart. If studies allowed for that factor, among others, and still showed an increase in cardiac problems among cannabis users, then cannabis would likely be a significant culprit.

If you have a cardiac condition, or any significant cardiac risk factors, use cannabis very cautiously, if at all, and work with your primary care physician, as well as with a cardiologist, if you have one, to maximize relief of pain, anxiety, and insomnia without worsening your cardiac condition with the use of cannabis or dangerous medications, such as NSAIDs.

The AHA (American Heart Association), like most professional medical organizations, tends to focus more on the harms of cannabis than on the clinical relief that people can receive from using it. Very few cardiologists treat patients with medical cannabis, so they might not be aware of its benefits to patients or how it can reduce the use of other drugs. They don't tend to factor in the cardiotoxic medications, such as NSAIDs, that patients might be using instead of cannabis—so I suspect that their pronouncements don't encompass the entire clinical picture. The AHA is clearly concerned about cannabis use. In one study the group concluded that "cannabis use is associated with adverse cardiovascular outcomes, with heavier use (more days per month) associated with higher odds of adverse outcomes."[3]

Once again, it is difficult to disentangle the significance of bad outcomes that are "associated" with cannabis use. Patients who are sicker than others, and who have more pain, insomnia, anxiety, and arthritis, are the ones who use cannabis. Another study reported that cannabis triggers heart attack, but mostly when it is smoked (which I also believe to be the case). These researchers' data showed that "like tobacco smoking, cannabis smoking may independently provoke MI [myocardial infarction]. Vaping and ingestion of cannabis might be less harmful, probably because absence of combustion prevents exposure to certain toxins in cannabis smoke, including carbon monoxide."[4]

As to whether cannabis causes or contributes to stroke, the data is also scattered. Just as with cardiac disease, it is likely that smoking cannabis contributes to stroke risk, due to the toxic combustion products. One study found that *any* marijuana use was linked with a higher risk of strokes, and people who used it most frequently had the highest odds. They also found that adults in the study who used marijuana daily had a 42 percent higher risk of stroke versus nonusers.[5] Again, this was an "associational" study, so it can't prove cause and effect, or directionality.

All that said, if you have risk factors for a stroke, or have had a stroke, I advise against smoking cannabis. I also advise approaching gummies and tinctures with caution, as they have not been proven to be safe (or dangerous, for that matter). Of course, untreated pain and anxiety aren't good for you either, so you must work with your doctor to decide which is the least harmful way to address your symptoms. For example, a modest dose of a gummy or an edible might be safer than NSAIDs or opioids.

For the sake of fairness, and to illustrate how conflicting the data can be, I will mention that other studies, such as the one below, show no increased risk of stroke or heart attack (although they found some association with adverse cardiovascular events in general).

> No statistically significant association was found between cannabis use and the risk of myocardial infarction compared to non-users. . . . Similarly, while the risk of stroke showed no significant association with cannabis use . . . a statistically significant association was observed between ever use of cannabis and the composite of any adverse cardiovascular events.[6]

In other words, cannabis use isn't associated with heart attack or stroke, but, confusingly, it is generally associated with the odds of a composite of adverse cardiac events. So . . . stay tuned! We need more research.

A recent concerning study aimed to evaluate the long-term cardiovascular effects of cannabis use in relatively healthy younger patients who were less than fifty years old. It showed an association between cannabis use and "adverse cardiovascular events, including MI [myocardial infarction], ischemic stroke [blockage or reduction of blood supply to the brain], HF [heart failure] and mortality."[7] Although this study shows only an association and doesn't demonstrate a causal link, it again raises the question of whether cannabis smoke helps trigger cardiac events.

In summary, if you have any risk factors for heart attack, arrhythmia, or stroke, please do not smoke cannabis and proceed cautiously with other cannabis formulations, such as edibles and tinctures. It is worth mentioning, in the context of contradictory data about cardiac events, that I have treated thousands of medical cannabis patients over the last quarter century, and not one of them has had a cardiovascular event that could be attributed to cannabis.

## PULMONARY EFFECTS

Cannabis use has not been definitively linked to the development of COPD, emphysema, or lung cancer. According to a prominent study, "Most cohort and case-control studies have failed to show that marijuana smoking is a significant risk factor for lung cancer despite the presence of procarcinogens in marijuana smoke."[8]

Components of marijuana smoke—such as tar, benzene, carbon monoxide, and polycyclic aromatic hydrocarbons—are known to cause cancer. Given that there are carcinogenic products in cannabis smoke, it can't possibly be healthy or safe to smoke cannabis. It is not impossible that heavy cannabis smoking will be linked to cases of lung cancer in the future, but to put it into context, smoking marijuana is significantly less dangerous than smoking cigarettes, which causes over 480,000 deaths per year, many of them from cancer.[9]

Doctors rarely recommend that people smoke cannabis as part of their medical routine to relieve symptoms, although that rule does not apply to chemotherapy, nausea, migraine, and end-of-life care. The dangers of smoking are a question of magnitude. It may not be particularly unhealthy to take a puff or two on the weekend, at a party, or out in the woods with friends but, on the other side of the spectrum, toking on your vape pen every ten minutes, sixty times a day, could be quite destructive to the lungs.

Smoked cannabis has been shown to cause symptoms of chronic bronchitis, including increased cough, sputum production, and wheezing. The smoke can be quite irritating to the lungs. Frequent cannabis smokers often have a "smoker's cough." Vape pens, which are made up of chemicals, are likely more harmful than joints or pipes. Whenever I have tried a vape pen, I wheezed for several minutes, and my lungs felt as if someone had gone over them with a buzz saw. That type of chronic inflammation and irritation can't possibly be good for your lungs.

Anyone who has *any* type of lung disease, such as COPD, should not be smoking cannabis, and should settle on another method of consumption (see chapter 2). People who smoke cigarettes or vape nicotine certainly shouldn't smoke or vape cannabis, as lung damage might worsen. Although it needs to be further studied, use of a dry herb vaporizer (see pages 30–32), which heats the cannabis flower into a vapor without actually burning it, may be significantly less harmful to the lungs. Several companies are working on safer smoking technology using a variety of filters, but it's not ready for showtime.

Many people decide to deny, minimize, or ignore the risks of smoking cannabis—and that is their choice. They shouldn't be bothered, criticized, or judged; smoking cannabis is a personal decision, as long as the smoke isn't harming or annoying anyone. Just like cigarettes, cannabis produces secondhand smoke that is not healthy for others to breathe in.

### CHS (Cannabis Hyperemesis Syndrome)

In the news these days, one hears more about an unpleasant and medically dangerous syndrome called cannabis hyperemesis syndrome, or CHS. In most circumstances, cannabis effectively helps alleviate nausea and vomiting, which is why people undergoing chemotherapy use it and why so many pregnant women are tempted to use it (even though this is not advised). Occasionally, people have a paradoxical reaction to medications, which means that the meds work in a manner opposite to that intended. For example, sometimes people take Benadryl or diphenhydramine (Tylenol PM) to help them sleep and find that it makes them wired and shaky instead. For a minority of heavy cannabis users, cannabis can have a paradoxical effect that causes severe nausea and vomiting—CHS. One can also experience acute nausea and vomiting from massive overconsumption of cannabis—it's called "greening out," and it is not pleasant to watch or experience.

CHS often requires a trip to the ER to help control symptoms and possibly a night or two in the hospital for intravenous medications, management of electrolytes, and administration of fluids. CHS usually doesn't respond to traditional medications for nausea, such as ondansetron (Zofran) or prochlorperazine (Compazine), which can make it incredibly challenging to treat. It often requires a heavy-handed pharmacological fix, such as using the antipsychotic haloperidol (Haldol). It has also been said that hot showers help alleviate CHS, although it is unclear why that might be the case. Some cannabis advocates believe that CHS is caused by a particular pesticide that is used in growing cannabis, but there is no evidence to support that assertion.

The only definitive treatment for CHS is to stop or, possibly, to drastically cut down on the use of cannabis. If you can't do that, you are likely dealing with cannabis addiction, which is best defined as continued use of cannabis despite negative consequences. If you experience severe nausea and vomiting, it is advisable to stop using cannabis immediately. If using it is very important to you, medically or otherwise, it is worth trying to substantially reduce the dose or to use a different ingestion method, to see if there is a way to consume cannabis without triggering CHS. In any case, it is best to work on this with your physician.

## DRIVING

The old joke is that when someone is drunk they will barrel through a red light, whereas if they are stoned on cannabis they carefully stop at a green light. All joking aside, it is strongly recommended that you do not drive for four hours after smoking or vaping cannabis and for eight hours after taking an edible or using a tincture. With cannabis use, the rate of motor vehicle accidents goes up, and driving skills go down. It is not safe to drive under the influence of cannabis.

As a primary care doctor, I am aware that people often drive after taking many of the medicines that I strongly advise them not to use before driving: If they are having an anxiety attack, they might take a benzodiazepine (Valium, Klonopin, Ativan) and then drive to the market or to work. If they are a construction worker, and their pain is bad enough, they might take an opioid before arriving at the construction site. Although people do this out of suffering and desperation to control symptoms, it can get them into a lot of trouble and also harm others. The same is true of driving under the influence of cannabis.

According to one study of cannabis and simulated driving in older adults, there was more weaving (or "standard deviation of lateral position") thirty minutes after the participants consumed cannabis.[10] Other studies have shown similar results. It can take longer to respond to traffic lights when under the influence of cannabis.

However, some experienced cannabis users think they are better drivers under the influence of cannabis because they drive more slowly and are extra-focused on safety concerns. It is true that stoned people tend to be much more aware of their impairment than drunk people. However, there is no evidence that using cannabis improves driving, under any circumstances. It is also true that people who drive under the influence tend to drive more slowly, which is one thing in their favor, although their reflexes might not be as sharp as they could be.

Several studies on cannabis-related driving impairment have found that people felt as if the effects of cannabis wore off several hours before their driving skills returned to normal. Thus, there was a temptation to drive even if they were still somewhat impaired, but did not think they were still impaired.[11] Very experienced cannabis users are likely to be less of a menace than people who aren't used to accommodating the effects of cannabis, but no one should be driving stoned.

All things being equal, cannabis doesn't raise the risk of a crash as much as alcohol. CBD by itself is typically not considered to be dangerous when you are driving or to increase the risk of an accident. However, if it makes you feel particularly sleepy, you should not drive.

## ACCIDENTAL OVERCONSUMPTION

For people of every age, emergency room visits are going up due to accidental exposure to cannabis. This occurs with both unintentional consumption and among people who unwittingly take too big a dose. There is concern among some that this issue is worsening with the legalization and availability of cannabis. I think overconsumption of cannabis is, in large part, due to a lack of education, but it hasn't helped that we formulate this strong medicine into succulent gummies and chocolates that any small child or pet, oblivious to the fact that they contain THC, would gladly eat. An unwitting adult could make the same mistake, thinking that such delicious-tasting edibles are just regular candy or misreading the label, and no wonder—these products are often not well marked. Labels should be clearer, and packaging should be more responsible and informative. Servings of gummies, for example, should be individually wrapped rather than loose in a bag. Just like gummies, the ten squares in big chocolate bars, each of which contains a substantial dose of THC, should be packaged individually.

Unsuspecting people, whether they are kids, adults, or elders, can get extremely ill if they overconsume cannabis (see pages 140–141 for issues involving the elderly). They can end up having a panic attack or a rapid heart rate, and wind up in the ER. Some of the products that are available in dispensaries are insanely potent and need to be labeled as such. They should also be displayed separately from other cannabis products.

We often recommend that people start with between 1 milligram and 2.5 milligrams of THC, to get used to the effect and avoid overshooting the proper dosage. My worst cannabis nightmare: I was once speaking to a group of addiction specialists at a cannabis dispensary, and I saw a candy bar with 1,100 milligrams of THC. Eating it would land almost anyone in the hospital. Each little square contained 110 milligrams of THC, which is more than enough to poison most people. I am experienced with cannabis, but if I had eaten just one of those 110-milligram chunks, I could have been sick for days. Ideally, when we legalize cannabis on a federal level, the entire industry should be more consistently regulated in terms of how products are labeled and packaged, to protect people from overly concentrated products.

The level of THC in cannabis flowers is extremely high these days, which can also lead to overconsumption. At parties, I have been called to assist baby boomers who took the same three bong hits they took in college, and then proceeded to utterly freak out, due to a cannabis overdose. Back in the day, cannabis was about 2–4 percent THC and now it is more than 20 percent THC. For that reason, those three bong hits were more like fifteen to twenty bong hits. People need to be educated about how incredibly strong modern cannabis products are and should be exceedingly careful about dosage. If you wish to smoke at a party, start with just one puff. You can always consume more later, but you can't undo what you've already consumed.

Some people compound the risk of accidental overconsumption by being irresponsible and not carefully storing cannabis products away from young children, teens, and pets. The best practice is not to buy cannabis in the form of candy or chocolate in homes with young people or animals. Instead, buy it in a form that looks and tastes like medicine, such as a pill or tincture. Most kids won't drink an unflavored, oily bottle of tincture. If you do buy candies, gummies, food products, or other treats that contain cannabis, it is imperative to store them with extreme care—out of harm's way—just as you would with other drugs and medicines. Do not keep them in the fridge or in kitchen cupboards or on countertops, and make sure they are very clearly marked, as they don't always come in packaging that clearly identifies the contents. If the label is missing from whatever the product is, you won't know how much THC it contains, or even that it contains THC in the first place. As it is, you can barely see the THC warning on many of the products sold in cannabis dispensaries. If you have teenagers at home, it would not be unreasonable to store cannabis products in a locked closet.

Unwittingly eating a cannabis-infused edible is the worst-case scenario for people because they don't know that they have been exposed to intoxicating THC and have no explanation or context for how impaired they might feel an hour later. Imagine if you were driving or caring for small children under those circumstances. The teenage daughter of a family I know left most of a strong cannabis chocolate bar on her dresser, and the person who helps clean the house ate it. She became profoundly ill before driving home. In this scenario, both the teenager and the person who helped herself to the chocolate were both at fault, but the real culprit was the unmarked bar of cannabis.

With better education and more responsible packaging of edibles (e.g., wrapping individual doses separately), I think we can minimize dangerous exposures. In Canada, for example, there are regulations for strict, sensible labeling and packaging of cannabis products and there's no reason we can't do the same in the US.

## MEDICATION INTERACTIONS

With CBD, there are more serious drug interactions than there are with regular THC/cannabis, although both can cause clinically significant drug interactions. There are fewer drug interactions with smoked cannabis, however, because THC goes directly into the bloodstream and doesn't get metabolized in the liver. If cannabis or CBD is taken as an edible or a tincture, which I recommend, as opposed to smoking it, one downside is that there is a greater potential for drug interactions.

According to a paper by Dr. Staci Gruber at Harvard's McLean Hospital, when CBD is ingested, it competes for the same liver enzymes that ordinarily metabolize and remove other drugs from the bloodstream: "CBD and other cannabinoids are metabolized extensively by the CYP450 system [of the liver], and also inhibit many of these enzymes, potentially leading to variable serum levels of other medications, as well as variable levels of cannabinoids when other medications modify the system."[12]

Interference of CBD with liver function can cause the level of other medications in your blood to rise or fall, which can lead to toxic effects or ineffective treatments. It is particularly important to keep an eye on drug interactions with medications, such as antiepileptics, immunosuppressants, and blood thinners, that need to be kept in a narrow range in the bloodstream. One study observed that "interactions between cannabis/cannabinoids and warfarin, valproate, tacrolimus, and sirolimus were the most widely reported and may pose the greatest risk to patients."[13] Drug interactions can go the other way, too. The medications you are taking can affect the levels of cannabis in the products you have consumed, which can make dosing more challenging.

CBD, in particular, has strong interactions with the liver. Typically, CBD increases the levels of other drugs in your system. For example, in a study titled "A Phase 1 Trial of the Pharmacokinetic Interaction Between Cannabidiol and Tacrolimus," the concurrent use of other drugs and CBD was shown to increase the level of tacrolimus (Prograf) by a factor of 4.2. Tacrolimus is an important medication for people who need to suppress their immune systems after an organ transplant, for example, so the level of tacrolimus must be stable and in range.[14]

CBD tends to interact with other medications at higher doses than most people typically take. For example, someone might take a 30-milligram gummy without experiencing any meaningful medication interactions. However, at higher doses, in the hundreds of milligrams, significant interactions are more likely. Many studies show that higher doses of CBD are more clinically effective. Lower-dose CBD products—which most people take—are less of a concern when it comes to medicine interactions, but they may also be less clinically effective.

CBD can directly affect and elevate one's liver enzymes, which is an indication of liver inflammation. This result has been seen, primarily, with very high doses of Epidiolex (an FDA-approved CBD-based medicine for childhood epilepsy), and is particularly true when Epidiolex is given along with other antiseizure medications, such as valproic acid. It is important to keep your doctor informed about your use of CBD, so that they can monitor your liver function.

Another type of drug interaction with cannabis has to do with anesthesia requirements. Chronic marijuana users can require more anesthesia,[15] which might increase the riskiness of the anesthesia. Cannabis users can, for example, require more sedation for endoscopies. Under no circumstances should you use cannabis on the day of your procedure or surgery. It is best to stop using it completely, if you can, several days or weeks beforehand. Cessation of use will also help you avoid withdrawal symptoms and drug interactions from cannabis while you are in the hospital.

Drug interactions with cannabis and CBD usually do not make it impossible for people to use these products. Rather, it is a question of clear communication between patient and doctor and, at times, more intensive clinical monitoring.

## ANXIETY

Although many people use cannabis to treat anxiety, some patients find the effects of cannabis to be anxiety-provoking. Cannabis is "biphasic" in regard to anxiety—in other words, it has two potential effects. In low doses, cannabis tends to lessen and alleviate anxiety. In high doses, however, it can worsen anxiety and even cause severe paranoia or psychotic symptoms. The challenge is that everyone has a different level of cannabis consumption at which their anxiety can be triggered, and they can transition from feeling relaxed to being anxious. In any case, one must be extremely careful, given the strength of cannabis these days. Some people may find that any amount of cannabis makes them paranoid. In that case, they may choose, rightly, to avoid it altogether. A lower dose of cannabis generally causes much less anxiety than a higher one. That is why we "start low and go slow" to get the right dose so that you won't overshoot and develop an uncomfortable symptom like anxiety. As people acclimate to the effects of cannabis and determine ideal dosage and delivery methods, anxiety often becomes less of an issue over time.

## ADDITIONAL RISKS TO OLDER PATIENTS

Older patients are at greater risk of harm than younger patients from use of virtually all medications and drugs, including cannabis and alcohol. This disparity is due to changes in our physiology as we age. Our liver and kidneys don't filter blood as efficiently as they once did. Drugs and medications, particularly cannabis, which is fat soluble, tend to stick around longer in our systems. Our brains are more sensitive to any potential damages—or side effects of medications—from traditional pharmaceuticals, as well as from cannabis and alcohol.

The vulnerability of older patients is especially significant when it comes to psychoactive drugs and medicines, which affect our mental processes, i.e., consciousness, mood, emotions, etc. Many substances, including cannabis, can lead to temporary problems with coordination, balance, and the ability to think clearly. Some of the worst culprits for older patients tend to be sedatives, sleep and anxiety medications, and painkillers—all of which can affect balance, mood, and cognition. Alcohol is often the most harmful in this regard, but cannabis can worsen the same problems, which is why it needs to be used cautiously, conservatively, and mindfully.

In older patients, there are specific risks and side effects to be concerned about, even with modest or occasional use of cannabis. Medical marijuana certainly doesn't help everyone. Some people can't tolerate it, even in low doses, perhaps because it makes them paranoid or sleepy, or maybe they just hate the way it makes them feel. Not least of all, cannabis can increase the risk of falls and accidents. Knowing about potential problems such as those will help you to recognize them and, hopefully, minimize or avoid them in the first place. As is true of all drugs and medications, there are safe and less safe ways to use cannabis. Knowledge is power, and the point of this book is to help you use cannabis safely, maximize the benefits, and minimize side effects.

## Cognition

One of the side effects of using cannabis is a significant, if temporary and reversible, decrease in short-term memory. For example, if you go to a party and take a puff or two of cannabis, you will probably remember who you spoke with, and that you had a good time, but you might not remember specific details about each conversation. This is a temporary effect, and after the cannabis wears off your memory will return to normal. However, that return might take longer for younger patients—adolescents, for example—if their use of cannabis is extremely heavy. It might also take longer for older patients, whose brains are more sensitive to cannabis. As a side note, facilitated forgetting (i.e., helpful loss of traumatic memories) is thought to explain, at least in part, how cannabis helps people with PTSD to overcome disruptive, intrusive memories (see chapter 4).

There is no good evidence suggesting that healthy adults who use cannabis are affected by long-term or permanent memory damage. However, one recent study, "Risk of Dementia in Individuals with Emergency Department Visits or Hospitalizations Due to Cannabis," showed that patients aged 45 to 104 whose hospital visits were related to cannabis were more likely to eventually develop a diagnosis of dementia.[16] The results of this study are not as severe as those related to the use of alcohol concerning the incidence of more dementia. Yet, it certainly suggests that the relationship between the use of cannabis and dementia needs to be studied more carefully. The likeliest explanation for the association the researchers found between cannabis and dementia is that people who have problems with cannabis (or alcohol) are generally less healthy than patients who don't have problems with either substance. As a consequence, the former type of users are more likely to encounter all types of health problems later in life, including dementia. Thus, a cannabis or alcohol problem could be an indicator of poor health. Alternatively, the findings could be due to some harmful effect of cannabis on our brains. We know that alcohol harms our brains, but this has not yet been seen to be the case with cannabis.

Temporary memory impairment caused by cannabis can be additive to any cognitive difficulties that a patient may already be struggling with. For example, if a patient has mild cognitive impairment, i.e., some loss of memory but not full dementia, the use of cannabis might make their memory worse until the effects wear off. There wouldn't be any permanent effect or worsening of memory. But if a patient uses medical cannabis every day for chronic pain, for example, their memory might be worse on those days. However, it might be less of a problem over time if they develop tolerance to the effects of cannabis.

Any loss of memory can be dangerous if a person is already struggling with cognitive impairment, whether it is age-related or a precursor to dementia. If a person's memory is even temporarily worsened (due to cannabis use, for example) on top of a chronic condition, the individual might be more likely to forget to turn off the stove or forget where they parked their car and get lost looking for it. If memory is impaired every day, due to cannabis use or anything else that might cause an impairment, you are, in essence, worsening the functioning of your memory—memory that you rely on for all of your everyday tasks. This is a problem that can be worsened by many medicines, such as those that are used to aid sleep and relieve pain, not just by cannabis.

Cannabis does not necessarily have an overall harmful effect on brain functioning. According to the work of Dr. Gruber (discussed in chapter 4), medical cannabis can improve the executive functioning of adult medical patients who need relief from pain or sleep disorders by lessening their need for opioids and sedatives and augmenting their participation in pleasurable activities. Some dementia patients improve symptomatically and behaviorally on CBD. Cannabis, or often just CBD, can help control their agitation and anxiety better than traditional pharmaceuticals, with fewer side effects. I have seen this in practice many times.

Interestingly, there is some evidence in mice that cannabis can protect memory as they age. The authors of one study found that "the endocannabinoid system (ECS) . . . modulates the physiological processes underlying aging." A low dose of THC reversed age-related decline in the cognitive performance of mice aged twelve and eighteen months.[17] So, if you have a pet mouse with dementia, consider giving it cannabis treats. Just kidding! As suggested, it's possible that cannabis might be able to reestablish cannabinoid signaling—an activity that could be related to the preservation of memory—in our aging brains. More research in this area needs to be done, as does targeted drug development.

The research done with mice needs to be applied to humans, so that we can see whether and how the different components of cannabis, or other aspects of the endocannabinoid system, might help with memory and age-related neurodegeneration. One interesting study in humans, which is consistent with the idea that cannabis might help preserve memory, reported that "men with a history of cannabis use had less cognitive decline from early adulthood to late midlife compared to men without a history of cannabis use. Among cannabis users, neither age of initiation of cannabis use nor frequent use was significantly associated with a greater age-related cognitive decline."[18]

That finding is intriguing and needs further study, but it shouldn't detract from the fact that cannabis can temporarily make short-term memory worse.

There is also speculation, and some research in animals, that suggests that CBD by itself might help protect memory by being neuroprotective.[19] CBD has an anti-inflammatory effect on certain critical cells in our brains that might be able to protect them from damage, but this is still under investigation (see chapter 7).

## Balance

Although balance can be impaired by many common medications for mood, pain, anxiety, sleep, epilepsy, allergies, blood pressure, bladder issues, etc., that is not necessarily a reason to avoid them. Instead, a prescribing physician must factor in issues with balance as a side effect, warn the patient—who, hopefully, can adjust and compensate for it—and monitor the clinical situation carefully. For example, I start older patients on blood pressure medications all the time and warn them to get up slowly—for the first few days after starting the medication—and to hold on to something, so that they don't fall. If loss of balance becomes a dangerous or intolerable side effect, the medicine needs to be changed.

Cannabis can negatively affect balance. One scenario that makes health care providers anxious is where a patient wakes up in the night to go to the bathroom and feels woozy, and trips and falls. That scenario can be particularly worrisome if the patient already has an unsteady gait, poor vison or coordination, or a history of falls; and it can be even more dangerous if the patient has just started using cannabis and is not used to the side effects.

Falls can partly be prevented with common-sense interventions, such as keeping the floor clear of things to trip over such as throw rugs or clutter, and using nightlights to clearly illuminate the pathway from the bed to the bathroom. Physical therapy can usually assist people with balance issues by helping them learn to get up slowly and take a moment to find their balance.

The results of one very small study of cannabis use in older adults, versus nonusers of the same age, indicate a higher fall risk, a poorer performance of balance while standing on one leg, and a slower gait. However, "no significant differences in cognitive function were found."[20]

Though not blameless, cannabis might not be as dangerous as other commonly used drugs in this regard. One study examined 36.7 million falls in patients aged sixty-five or older and reported that "prevalences of specific substances detected were 9.3 percent for benzodiazepines, 4.3 percent for cannabinoids, 8.0 percent for ethanol, and 15.0 percent for opioids."[21] In other words, the worst culprits for falls during the night were opioids, followed by benzodiazepines (Valium, Klonopin, Ativan), then alcohol, and, finally, lower down but still significant, cannabis. Cannabis is less likely to lead to falls than many of the medications it can replace, but nonetheless, it was implicated in 4.3 percent of falls, a very serious side effect that patients must be counseled on. Gabapentinoids, such as gabapentin (Neurontin) and pregabalin (Lyrica), which are commonly prescribed pain medications, have been associated with a doubling of hip fractures due to falls.[22] This has not been shown to be the case with cannabis, which may prove to be a safer option than some medications, even if it is not entirely safe.

## Dizziness

The word "dizzy" can mean several different things: vertigo, when it feels like the room is spinning, or wooziness, a sensation of lightheadedness. As a primary care provider, I frequently try to disentangle what my patients are feeling when they say, "I am dizzy."

For patients who use cannabis and complain of feeling dizzy, I have to determine whether they're feeling that way from the cannabis—because dizziness is a common side effect of THC—or simply voicing that they are high or stoned—an effect that is sought after by recreational users, but met with mixed opinions by medical users.

If patients complain about dizziness after cannabis use, it must be taken extremely seriously, even if we aren't always sure what "dizzy" means. An Israeli study found that "dizziness" was the most common side effect experienced by older medical cannabis patients, with 9.7 percent experiencing dizziness as a side effect.[23] I have treated patients with lightheadedness from cannabis and a few patients with true vertigo. In the elderly, both can increase the risk of falls. I had one patient whose vertigo got profoundly worse after he used cannabis. Unfortunately, for an unknown reason, he had decided to use a vastly higher dose than I suggested, but neither of us wished to restart cannabis consumption after the vertigo worsened, and he had to stop using it entirely.

If you are experiencing vertigo, you should stop using cannabis altogether. If you feel lightheaded, you might try to significantly lower the dose and see whether it is effective without causing dizziness.

### Syncope/Loss of Consciousness

"Syncope" is defined as an abrupt loss of consciousness. Several medical conditions can cause syncope, such as severe dehydration or cardiac problems, including arrhythmia, which cannabis can bring on in some people. Cannabis can also cause syncope, but it is a rare side effect. I know of several patients who have suffered from cannabis-induced syncope, which generally occurs after an inexperienced user inadvisedly takes a huge puff, or several puffs of cannabis, and down they go.

I was once asked, with some urgency, to help someone with this condition at a New Year's party at my friend's house. A woman in her late sixties had decided to smoke cannabis after not using it for several decades. She took a few huge puffs (of cannabis that is much stronger than it used to be), which is not at all what I would have recommended. She became extremely anxious and passed out. At that point, another friend ran into the room and said, "Pete—you're the only doctor here who isn't stoned, and we have an emergency." I made sure she was okay, monitored her, and called 911. After a few minutes she woke up. She was evaluated at the hospital and found to be no worse for wear, but the episode was extremely scary for her and for us, as well.

If a patient experiences syncope after using cannabis, they should have a complete medical workup to make sure that it didn't trigger or uncover a dangerous underlying condition, such as an arrhythmia. They likely shouldn't use cannabis again, unless they wish to drastically readjust their dosage downward to be on the safe side, and carefully experiment with it under controlled circumstances, e.g., sitting in a chair at home with other people not using cannabis, not carousing at a party.

## Dry Mouth

In the study cited above, 7.1 percent of patients treated with cannabis experienced dry mouth. Though it's not the most ominous side effect, dry mouth can be uncomfortable, at the very least. It can also impair speech by reducing saliva production, and can harm the health of our teeth by impacting enamel erosion and gum disease. Many commonly prescribed medications, such as amitriptyline and trazodone, or Benadryl, can also cause dry mouth. I once tried trazodone for insomnia and couldn't believe how bad the dry mouth symptoms were. I could barely talk the next day. It felt as if my mouth were stuffed with cotton balls. That side effect certainly isn't specific to cannabis, but it can cause a profound case of dry mouth, especially when smoked.

Dry mouth can also cause people to drink too many liquids and then need to go to the bathroom a lot during the middle of the night, which can disrupt sleep and lead to falls.

## Psychosis

Several substances can cause a transitory psychosis called "substance-induced psychosis." Transitory psychoses are characterized by symptoms such as delusions, hallucinations, paranoia, and disorganized thinking. They are extremely troubling, are disruptive, and can last from days to months after the "substance" was ingested. Many medications, including steroids, alcohol, amphetamines—such as methylphenidate (Ritalin and Concerta) or Adderall for ADHD—cannabis, and psychedelics, which are increasingly popular, can cause this (see chapter 9). Cannabis is the drug that most commonly causes substance-induced psychosis, however, and although it largely affects people in their twenties and thirties, it can affect anyone at any age.

Substance-induced psychosis is an extremely serious condition and entails entering a dangerous psychotic state for days or weeks until it resolves with antipsychotic medications and supportive care.

If you have a history of any type of psychosis, especially substance-induced psychosis from cannabis, I strongly recommend that you consider abstaining completely from cannabis. In addition to causing psychosis, cannabis can destabilize people who have recovered, or who are currently stabilized, from a psychotic disorder earlier in life, such as schizophrenia or bipolar disorder.

## Accidents and Injuries

Any drug, including cannabis, that impairs your ability to think and perceive clearly, can increase your chances of accidents and injuries. It bears repeating that people shouldn't drive or operate heavy machinery under the influence of cannabis. They should be particularly careful when crossing streets, riding bicycles, or doing other activities that can involve accidents. Obviously, they should not use firearms.

## Cannabis Overdose

There has been an increase in cannabis poisonings and overdoses in the elderly as more people use cannabis—medically and otherwise. Edibles are largely involved because it is all too easy for people to accidentally take too large a dose or unwittingly consume an unmarked product. Cannabis-related hospital visits are increasing among adults over sixty-five, one study indicated. The study also acknowledged that this "under-recognized at-risk group" needs more in the way of "prevention and intervention" when it comes to using cannabis.[24]

I agree with providing prevention and intervention—especially education—and better regulation and packaging of edibles, so that people don't consume too much.

A cannabis overdose (or cannabis poisoning) is medically dangerous, but it is not as immediately life-threatening as an overdose of opioids or alcohol. Cannabis overdoses can cause a panic attack and put an enormous amount of stress on your heart, possibly triggering an arrhythmia or even a heart attack. Symptoms of an overdose can include racing heart, anxiety, panic attacks, palpitations, transient psychosis, extreme confusion, delusions, hallucinations (although rarely), and nausea/vomiting ("greening out"—see page 123).

It is profoundly unpleasant and scary to go through an overconsumption event with cannabis. I would like to re-emphasize that overconsumption of cannabis must be scrupulously avoided. Avoiding an accidental overdose is why we constantly nag new cannabis patients about starting low and going slow. The goal is to reach but not overshoot a helpful dosage. As with all medications, the aim is to use the lowest effective dose.

Most cannabis users have accidentally overconsumed cannabis at some point. Experienced users often deal with an episode of overconsumption on their own, by acquiring emotional support; hydrating; and sitting in a calm, quiet space. However, if you feel any heart palpitations or chest pain, or your anxiety continues to rise, despite your being in a calm environment, the ER is likely the right place for you. There, you can be watched closely—your vital signs will be monitored and, if you need one, you'll be given a sedative. Taking the right dose of cannabis, and not too high a dose, requires planning and careful attention to detail, because cannabis is much stronger than it used to be. I can't emphasize that enough. It is best to work with a cannabis specialist or a doctor who is educated on how to advise patients to use cannabis safely.

A cannabis overdose can happen in a variety of ways—although edibles are usually the culprit. The one time I experienced an accidental overconsumption was in the context of a very common scenario: My friends were making marijuana brownies. This is a cautionary tale. When baking marijuana brownies, or cookies, do not freely consume the batter, no matter how good it tastes! Hanging out with friends to bake regular brownies might be an enjoyable activity, but it can rapidly become miserable if the batter is cannabis-infused. There is no way to track the dose when eating batter, and it's difficult to stop eating it once you start. It made me extremely ill, with nausea, anxiety, and palpitations, for hours, until the cannabis wore off; it was an experience I will never repeat.

Another distressingly common scenario that can result in overconsumption involves gummies, chocolates, and other edibles. A common rookie mistake is to take an edible and then forget that there is a time delay before you feel any effect. With an edible, the cannabis doesn't kick in for forty-five to ninety minutes. After half an hour, people say, "Nothing happened; maybe I need some more." They then consume a few more edibles and . . . an hour later, when all the edibles are fully absorbed, they have consumed double or triple the intended dose. This never ends well.

As I keep noting, smoked flower is extremely strong today, compared to how it used to be in the 1960s and 1970s, with THC levels that routinely rise above 20 percent. If you smoke cannabis, start with just one small puff and then wait a few minutes to see how high you are and if your symptoms are relieved. You can always take a second puff.

## Tips for Using Medical Cannabis Safely and Effectively

We are still learning how to minimize the harms that may affect older people who use cannabis. The effects on the elderly haven't been extensively studied. Most of the research on cannabis has been conducted on teenagers and younger adults. This is due, in part, to stigma about older people using medical cannabis, as well as to, possibly, some institutional ageism. As the rates of cannabis use in the elderly continue to grow, more research will certainly be conducted. Here are some tips though to help if you are considering using medical cannabis:

- **Work with a doctor** who has experience advising patients on the use of medical cannabis, as well as of CBD. They can advise you on how to get started on proper dosing and other safety issues. They can also follow your progress and adjust your regimen as needed. You might need to consult with a cannabis specialist if your doctor doesn't feel comfortable with this issue. Some physician cannabis specialists haven't practiced mainstream medicine for a long time. They just prescribe cannabis. Try to pick a cannabis specialist who is also currently practicing medicine, so they are up to date on all the latest medical information. There are a lot of quacks out there.
- **Start low and go slow!** A huge dose of cannabis is a recipe for disaster, especially if you're just starting out. Try to have some idea of what you want before going to the dispensary, so you don't get upsold and end up taking stronger products than you want. (See chapter 6 about going to a dispensary.) Never take an edible if you don't know the dosage, even if your kids or a close friend gave it to you.
- **Always go through the legal system,** where cannabis is regulated by the state. It can be tempting to ask family members to purchase products from the illicit market because it is much less expensive. The extra cost of buying cannabis legally, due to regulations and taxes, pays for a tremendous amount of safety monitoring. This is the best way to know exactly what you are getting in the products you buy (e.g., how much THC and other components they contain), as well as what you aren't getting (mold, pesticides, heavy metals). It also helps the state generate vitally needed tax revenue.
- **Be open with your health care providers,** personal aides (if you have them), and family members about your

medical cannabis use, so that they can be on the lookout for potential side effects.

- **Be particularly careful of maintaining your balance** while walking or moving around in general, particularly when you've just started using cannabis or when you increase the dose. People tend to get used to slightly higher levels of cannabis with a subtle increase in the dose, but during the time immediately after changing the dose, be extra vigilant.
- **If you are having uncomfortable symptoms,** such as wooziness, confusion, dry mouth, or any cardiac symptoms, let your doctor or cannabis specialist know immediately.
- **If you can avoid it, don't smoke cannabis**—use one of the other consumption methods discussed in chapter 2, to spare your lungs and, in all likelihood, your heart.
- **If you start having severe anxiety,** ask someone to sit with you until you feel better. If your anxiety becomes extreme or is accompanied by chest pain, have someone take you to the ER, or call 911.

## WHO SHOULD GENERALLY AVOID CANNABIS?

- **Teenagers.** Please tell your grandkids to knock it off with the weed. Don't encourage them to use it—even if it seems like something you can bond over. Try not to use it around them and to keep it out of sight and smell when they come to visit. Keep your cannabis locked up or hidden away. You can discuss this with them openly if the subject comes up.

Physicians and cannabis experts are wary of teens using cannabis. There are concerns that when cannabis is used heavily and very early in life (e.g., by age sixteen) it could impact future brain development. I typically advise teens to wait until they're at least eighteen years old, although the later they start using cannabis the better. Exceptions include teens who are undergoing chemotherapy or being treated with CBD for autism spectrum disorder.

- **Pregnant and breastfeeding women.** The concern is that using cannabis while pregnant or breastfeeding can affect fetal outcomes. THC crosses the placenta and concentrates in breast milk. This means that if you use cannabis while pregnant or breastfeeding, your fetus or infant is exposed to THC, which can affect their newly developing brains and bodies. Unfortunately, the data on this subject is contradictory and inconclusive, because it is unethical to experiment directly on pregnant women. You can't just give a thousand women cannabis and see if it results in birth defects.

To be safe, I recommend that women abstain from cannabis during pregnancy and breastfeeding. An exception might be made if there is no other safe alternative for treating symptoms. For example, both cannabis and traditional pharmaceuticals are usually effective in treating morning sickness, but if it becomes severe (a condition called hyperemesis gravidarum), doctors quickly escalate the use of pharmaceuticals. Under those circumstances, it is not unreasonable to ask whether cannabis might be safer or more dangerous to use than stronger pharmaceuticals—none of which are entirely safe during pregnancy. Truthfully, we don't know how dangerous cannabis is during pregnancy, because studies have focused predominantly on women who use illegal smoked cannabis. If cannabis is legal and regulated, and isn't smoked, it may turn out to be not particularly harmful.

- **People with a personal or family history of any type of psychosis, including schizophrenia and bipolar disorder.** Cannabis use can destabilize people, especially younger people, who have these illnesses—and it can contribute to them in the first place. Usually, if a psychotic illness is going to declare itself, it does so in one's twenties or thirties, so most older patients should be in the clear and probably won't develop a new psychotic disorder, such as schizophrenia or bipolar disorder. A person who has a diagnosis of any type of psychotic disease may wish to refrain from using cannabis, for fear of becoming destabilized. Of course, destabilization is less likely if the disorder has been dormant for decades.
- **People with unstable cardiac conditions or risk factors for those conditions.** Depending on the dosage, as well as on the user's experience with cannabis, using it can raise heart rate and blood pressure. In doses that are too high, or in people who are vulnerable, using cannabis can cause severe anxiety, which, in turn, can significantly increase heart rate. If you have a tendency toward, or a history of, arrhythmia or coronary events, or risk factors for a stroke, cannabis could trigger or exacerbate those conditions. Smoking cannabis is more dangerous than other consumption methods due to its combustion products and the temporary bronchial inflammation it can cause. Data on this issue is somewhat contradictory (see chapter 5), and some people with cardiac conditions can nonetheless benefit from cannabis—albeit with careful use.
- **People with lung disease, such as emphysema or COPD, or any active respiratory infection (including Covid).** Smoking cannabis can only irritate symptoms of these conditions. It can make lung disease, or the inflammation of one's lungs, worse. Although cannabis has never been

implicated in the development of COPD or lung cancer, cannabis smoke contains some ugly combustion products that are best avoided. Responsible doctors never recommend smoking cannabis, except for some specific indications discussed in chapter 4 (e.g., terminal cancer, chemotherapy, migraine).

- **People who have had a bad reaction to cannabis.** As with any other drug, you must either stop using cannabis immediately or use it with extreme caution if you've had a bad reaction to it in the past. Some examples of bad reactions include panic attacks, allergic reactions (rare), anxiety or otherwise freaking out, hallucinations, passing out (syncope), dizziness, vomiting, falls, palpitations or heart attack, or just feeling crummy. Some people do not like the feeling of being high and never get used to it, while others, who may have had a bad reaction to a very high dose of smoked cannabis in college, might elect to try a much smaller dose of a legal, regulated edible or tincture and see if they have better luck.
- **People with a history of addiction to other drugs.** It is debatable whether people who were previously addicted to other drugs, such as opioids or alcohol, are more likely to develop a problem with cannabis *or* whether cannabis can generally support and aid recovery from those addictions. I suspect the latter is true and have written on the topic extensively. In any case, proceed with caution if you have been addicted to other drugs, such as opioids or alcohol. Pay attention to your usage pattern and make sure that the dose and frequency aren't drastically escalating. If you have been diagnosed with a severe cannabis addiction, you must find a way to stop using cannabis. Medical professionals can often help with this.

Other reasons some people need to stop consuming medical cannabis might include: loss of the drug's effectiveness, its unaffordability, a new job with an upcoming drug test, or a move to a state or country where cannabis is not legally available.

If a patient has had a dangerous reaction to cannabis, such as psychosis or arrhythmia, they must stop using cannabis immediately, even if doing so is uncomfortable. Patients who are trying to transition away from cannabis should usually be encouraged to gradually taper the dosage in order to avoid withdrawal symptoms. Those symptoms can be difficult and often include insomnia; poor appetite; irritability; and weird, vivid dreams. Withdrawal symptoms typically last a week or two and, although they may be unpleasant, they are not dangerous.

CHAPTER 6

# What Are the Practicalities of Using Medical Cannabis?

In states where cannabis is legal, you can't just buy it at the supermarket or at your local pharmacy. Cannabis is sold in specific, highly regulated locations, which are called dispensaries, of which there are three types:

1. **A recreational dispensary** is a store, located in a state where recreational marijuana is legal, and in which any adult over the age of twenty-one can purchase various cannabis products, such as flower, edibles, and tinctures.
2. **A medical dispensary** is oriented toward providing patients with medical marijuana products. To enter a medical dispensary and purchase products, you must have a medical marijuana card that your doctor can provide. (Information about how to procure a medical marijuana card is covered in this chapter.)
3. **A mixed-use dispensary** sometimes caters to both medical and recreational patients at the same time. This chapter is meant to explain and demystify the experience of purchasing cannabis products.

## WHAT IS IT LIKE GOING INTO A DISPENSARY?

Even before you walk into a dispensary, you can get a good idea of what to expect and what you might buy, once you get there, by taking a look at their product menu, which is usually posted online. Viewing the menu can help you narrow down the options. You can even look at the menu with your doctor or cannabis specialist to help you wade through a raft of products that can be overwhelming.

Going to a cannabis dispensary, at least in the states where I've visited them, is a very different experience than going to a liquor store or smoke shop. Dispensaries tend to be much nicer. When you first arrive, you must immediately show your ID to a person at a desk, just to get through the front door. (Often, you'll see a security guard sitting out front, looking bored out of their mind.) At cannabis dispensaries, everyone is checked upon entry. Even if you are a hundred years old, you will be carded. If you have a medical marijuana card, you can show it as well (if you are in a medical marijuana dispensary and not just a recreational one, that is). You will also need to show your ID upon purchasing items, so keep it handy. Note that you cannot bring children or teens to a dispensary, as you can to a liquor store: Only adults over the age of twenty-one, and who have proper identification, will be admitted.

Once your ID has been scanned, you'll be buzzed through locked doors and enter a spacious, spa-like room. Just like other retailers, dispensaries can vary greatly in quality and decor. Many of them are tastefully decorated and welcoming, with fancy lighting and sparkling displays, in an ongoing attempt to destigmatize cannabis use. Other customers will span an incredible range of ages, from twenty-one-year-olds to octogenarians.

As you enter the dispensary, you'll notice that the walls are lined with shelves crammed with paraphernalia, such as pipes, rolling papers, vaporizers, lighters, and containers for storing cannabis. Next, you'll get in line in front of a central counter, where the weed is sold, under a large menu of offerings. When it is your turn, go up to the counter to discuss what you wish to purchase with the budtender, the knowledgeable person behind the counter, who will help you find and purchase the right products for you.

Each dispensary handles the way it showcases and sells products a little differently. Most dispensaries exhibit their various products in glass display cases—and some let you smell and even touch samples of the cannabis flower. Then, using an electronic screen, you can order what you want, pay for your purchases at the counter, and be on your way. If this process is confusing for you, people are readily available to help you, including budtenders who can give you recommendations about what to purchase. Don't forget to ask about discounts.

When you get to the counter at the dispensary, you must pay for your purchases with cash. Most will also accept bank cards, but it is important to check beforehand. Many dispensaries have cash machines outside the stores, which may charge a small fee. Dispensaries do not accept credit cards because of the ongoing federal illegality of cannabis, which, in turn, makes the use of credit cards to purchase cannabis illegal. In the eyes of the federal government, selling cannabis is still like a drug deal, which frightens the credit card companies. At some point, when sensible legislation allows the cannabis industry to access banking services, the credit card situation will get better.

Once you have made your purchase, the product will be put into a nondescript bag so that you can leave the store discreetly. Nevertheless, if your neighbors and acquaintances happen to see you as you are leaving a cannabis dispensary with your nondescript bag, they will likely put two and two together.

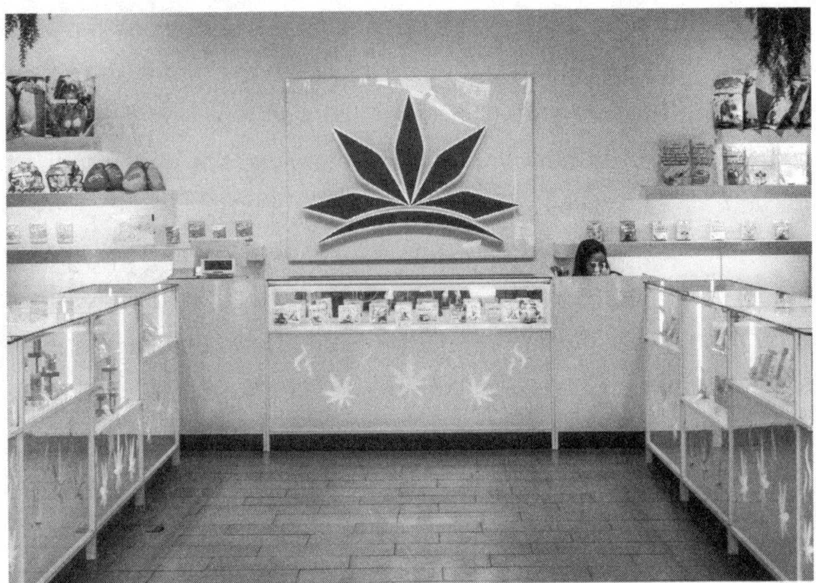

**Cannabis dispensaries are the state-regulated outlets where both medical and recreational cannabis are sold.**

## Finding the Right Strain

One overwhelming aspect of going to a dispensary is the wide variety of brands, strains, and consumption methods for different types of marijuana. Consequently, it can be intimidating and difficult to know what to buy. Looking at the dispensary menu can be confusing, too, when it offers things like "Durbin Poison," "Orange Tangie," and many other strains of cannabis that will likely mean nothing to you, especially if you're a newcomer. There are now thousands of different strain names, making it difficult to know what to purchase if you haven't researched them in advance. Even if you believe, as I do, that some of the differences between strains are exaggerated, it can still be difficult to know what to order, simply because there are so many options. Each dispensary in your town may have unique strains as well, as there is little consistency or standardization across the industry.

In fact, most strain names usually don't signify very much and are vaguely classified into "indica" and "sativa" (see page 69), even though there has been no meaningful botanical difference between the strains for decades.[1] An indica is supposed to be relaxing ("in da couch") and a sativa is supposed to be helpful with energy and focus, but, again, those distinctions are vague and not particularly helpful. Most of what you get is a hybrid of the two strains, with qualities of both types, regardless of what the label might say. Strains can have some minor differences, however. Generally, I interpret the word "indica" to mean a strain that someone, at some point, found relaxing, and "sativa" to denote a type that someone found energizing, even though the words are modern-day surrogates for what was once a real botanical distinction between the strains.

Furthermore, a strain (e.g., "Sour Diesel") in one place can have a totally different chemical makeup when sold under the same name at another location. "Sour Diesel" in Boston is completely different from "Sour Diesel" in San Francisco, and to make things even more confusing, there can also be differences in chemical makeup from store to store within the same town or city. There is very little regulation or standardization of any of this. People can claim whatever they want to about various strains, but invariably it boils down to advertising. In Israel and elsewhere, of late, there has been some interesting research into the possibility of developing different types of cannabis that can address various medical conditions or symptoms—an intriguing proposition, but one that hasn't been borne out yet by science.

As useful as it is to understand what the subtle differences are between strains, the more important consideration for medical patients is the percentage of THC, the percentage of CBD, and the major "minor" components in the strain, such as other cannabinoids and terpenes (see chapter 2). The information on the label—specifically the chemical components in the cannabis—is infinitely more important than the name of the strain or the store's description of it. That said, if you find a strain that works for you, stick with it. Some trial and error never hurts when it comes to finding a product that works best for you. This can be done with the help of a journal, where you can write down what you tried and what the effects were.

For more money, you can even buy a celebrity brand of cannabis, which is generally no different than the generic brand—you're just paying a premium for the association with the celebrity. In the supermarket, you can buy name brand-name foods or the generic versions, which cost less. Often, those products come from identical manufacturers. The same general idea is largely true of weed, although the genetics of the plant can vary.

You also can pay for an app on your phone that supposedly links your medical condition to a particular strain or product. These apps are a massive scam that just make money for the businesspeople and the dispensaries that run them. There isn't any good science to back up these products, and they take advantage of the fact that people don't always know what to buy.

So, how does one wade through all of this nonsense with strains and figure out what to buy?

First, try different strains, and if you find one that works for you, stick with it. You can also ask the budtenders which strain might be uplifting, for energy and focus, or relaxing and sedating, say, for sleep, pain, or anxiety control—if that is what you are looking for. Ask friends or family members what works best for them. There are also many patient support groups and online discussions that might give you some suggestions.

## Deciphering Labels

When you're shopping at a dispensary, labels on the products you want to buy should clearly indicate how much THC and CBD they contain. Increasingly, the labels include ingredients other than THC and now let us know which other minor cannabinoids (e.g., CBC, CGB, CBN) and terpenes are in the mix (see chapter 2). As customers get more savvy and educated, and as the industry does a better job with labeling, we'll learn more about the different components of cannabis and, consequently, get better at predicting the effects of different types of cannabis and how they might best alleviate our symptoms.

In their current incarnation, however, the labels—and the labs that test cannabis products—are not consistently well-regulated by the states, which means that products might not be accurately labeled. Some cannabis companies do "lab shopping" to find a lab that gives them the specific results they are looking for (very high THC, for example), which they can then advertise on the label. This practice shouldn't be legal. Going forward, with better regulation of all aspects of the cannabis industry, labeling practices should improve. Even with accurate labels, however, very few people know enough about the different components of cannabis to predict the likely effects of minor cannabinoids and terpenes. That situation will change for both patients and recreational users as product labels become more transparent and as all of us learn more about cannabis.

## Flower

Once you have navigated the bewildering number of, and names for, the different strains of cannabis flower, and you have decided which ones you want to try, you are ready to buy. How much do you buy? Making that decision can be bewildering as well.

The amount of flower in containers ranges from a gram (enough roughly for two joints), to an eighth of an ounce (3.5 grams, which is enough for seven to nine joints), to an entire ounce. You can buy little cannisters or bags of the dried flower, which can be ground up for smoking, cooking, or placing in a dry herb vaporizer. If you prefer to smoke cannabis flower and want more convenience than comes with rolling your own joints, you can buy pre-rolled joints, which cost more per amount of cannabis than they would if you rolled your own. You can also put cannabis flower into a pipe, which can also be purchased in a dispensary or smoke shop.

A grinder for cannabis flower is often useful, regardless of whether you are smoking it, putting it in a dry herb vaporizer, or cooking with it. The smaller, ground-up particles have more surface area to extract the cannabinoids and they burn or cook more efficiently.

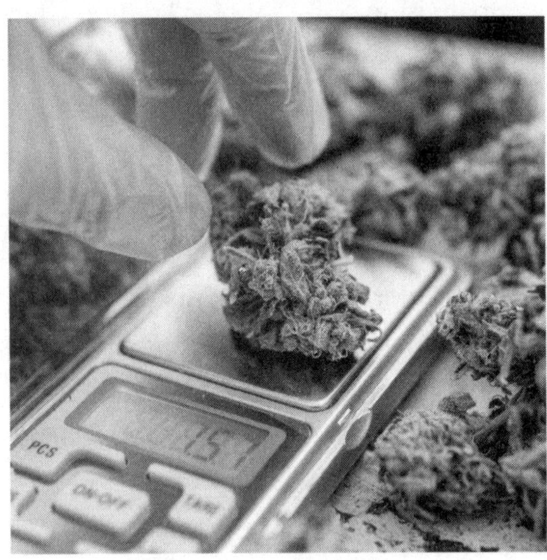


**At cannabis dispensaries, cannabis flower is sold by weight.**

## A Note on Budtenders

The budtenders who work behind the counter at dispensaries are among the nicest people you will ever meet. They tend to be cannabis enthusiasts who are excited to be working in an industry they believe in, and that is finally legal and accessible. They are often eager to provide recommendations about strains and products for symptoms that might be troubling you, which can be very helpful, because, as I've mentioned, it can be so difficult to wade through dozens of different strains without some guidance.

But—bear in mind that budtenders aren't medically trained. In fact, they are trained very minimally, if at all, and should not be making medical recommendations. If a budtender says something along the lines of "For lupus, the strain 'Space Alien' is the best one to treat your immune system," that recommendation is wholly inappropriate. On the other hand, a budtender might reasonably say, "For chronic pain, other customers have found 'Space Alien' to be helpful." That would be the safer recommendation, because the budtender is just sharing their experience with treating symptoms—not giving medical advice.

Having said all that, it can be very helpful to have some idea of what you are looking for before you go to a dispensary. For some people, looking into different types of cannabis becomes an interesting new hobby that they discuss with friends and fellow patients. Ask your cannabis doctor, friends, and other patients for suggestions. I've found that many seniors first try cannabis on the recommendation of their adult children, so don't hesitate to ask them for suggestions, but although their ideas about what to use are often spot on, they can be less than ideal if the composition and dose of the cannabis is not appropriate for older users. The most important thing to focus on is the amount of CBD and THC—and, potentially, any other components of cannabis, such as the other minor cannabinoids—that you might want. You can then decide how you wish to consume it (as an edible, a tincture, a topical, etc.). Some states require pharmacists to work in dispensaries, which is helpful, since they can provide an on-site source of medical competence, help prevent unwanted drug interactions, and advise patients on what types of marijuana might be helpful for particular conditions.

### Other Products

See chapter 2 for a comprehensive list of all the cannabis products you might find at a dispensary, including skin patches, suppositories, seltzers, mints, lozenges, and throat sprays.

As you purchase cannabis products, you'll need to decide which paraphernalia, if any, you need to comfortably consume those products. Dispensaries are chock-full of paraphernalia, and it can be intimidating to behold the myriad accessories that cannabis consumers use. Do you need a pipe? Rolling papers? A lighter? A dry herb vaporizer? Each modality has its own advantages and limitations. Some methods of consumption, such as inhaling, allow cannabis to kick in quickly and provide rapid relief, while others, such as edibles, might take longer to take effect, but provide longer-lasting relief. Having a basic understanding of the different ways to consume medical cannabis can go a long way toward effectively alleviating symptoms and minimizing side effects.

Or maybe you are content to just eat edibles or use tincture under your tongue—neither of which requires any additional purchases.

## MEDICAL CANNABIS CARD

As noted earlier, as of this writing, medical cannabis is legal in thirty-nine states. There are medical cannabis programs in each of them, including twenty-five states where cannabis is legal for recreational use as well. These programs give patients perks, such as paying lower taxes on cannabis products and getting preferential treatment in some dispensaries.

## Benefits of Getting a Medical Cannabis Card

- **Medical advice:** The process of getting a medical cannabis card presents a wonderful opportunity to consult with a knowledgeable doctor or, in some states, a nurse. This process allows you to get helpful suggestions on usage, dose, drug interactions, potential adverse reactions, and delivery mechanisms. This situation is vastly preferable to getting your medical card at a more corporate "card mill," where you pay a fee and are given a card without learning much about how to use cannabis safely and effectively.
- **Tax break:** Most states will give you a large tax break on the cannabis products you buy with a medical cannabis card, which can help you save a substantial amount of money over time, particularly if you use a significant amount of cannabis. For example, in Massachusetts, a medical card exempts you from paying the 20 percent tax that you'd ordinarily have to pay with the purchase of recreational cannabis. That means you can save $20 for every $100 of product you buy.
- **Discounts:** Many dispensaries have "new patient specials" for people who have new medical cannabis cards. In addition to not having to pay the tax, you can also get large discounts. At some dispensaries in Massachusetts, you get $50 off for every $50 you spend, up to $200 dollars. Add that to not paying the 20 percent tax, and you can make out very well.
- **VIP treatment:** Some dispensaries give special treatment, put people in a faster line, and reserve or prioritize products for medical patients who have a medical cannabis card.
- **Drug tests:** If you are employed, and your employer requires you to take a drug test, a medical card can potentially protect you. In some, but not all, situations, your employer can waive a positive test because it has been medically justified by a

physician. This is currently not the case, however, for some safety-sensitive jobs—for example if you're a pilot or work for the US government, which are jobs that don't allow exemptions. In fact, if you work for any arm of the government, say the Department of Defense, you can't use medical cannabis, unless you wish to assume the risk of getting caught and fired.

- **Pain or addiction clinics:** A medical cannabis card can help you if you are a patient at a pain clinic or an addiction clinic. Some of these clinics test for cannabis and can get upset with you for using medical cannabis (which they don't necessarily view as helpful). A medical card legitimizes your use. Some clinics will kick you out for cannabis use, which is unfair and unhelpful, but medical cards are becoming increasingly useful in those situations.
- **Growing cannabis:** In many states a medical card allows you to grow your own cannabis at home, which is less expensive than buying it from a retailer—and it can become a fun, wholesome hobby. When growing cannabis, you can do the basics and just watch it grow, or you can get into the science of it and fine-tune different parameters such as moisture, nutrients, and light.

One warning for gun owners: You aren't allowed to possess a medical cannabis card and a gun license at the same time. People are forced to choose between their guns and their legal weed, although I expect this will change at some point.

## How to Get a Medical Cannabis Card

To get a medical cannabis card, you must meet with a specialized doctor or, in some states, a nurse, who is certified to give you a card. Ideally, in addition to filling out the paperwork, they will teach you a good deal about how to use cannabis and what to watch out for. In a perfect world, your own primary care doctor, oncologist, or pain specialist would know how to do this. Thankfully, this is increasingly the case as doctors get up to speed on medical cannabis. Your overall care will be more coherent if cannabis care is done by one of your regular doctors.

Alternatively, you can go to a cannabis specialist who may know all about cannabis but know nothing about your regular care, your medications, or your specialists. Under those circumstances, it is best to provide them with as much accurate information as possible because they may not have access to your electronic medical records. Be aware that some cannabis specialists haven't practiced regular medicine in years, and are rusty at best, so as noted earlier, it is better to see a cannabis specialist who is currently practicing regular medicine as well.

The least effective way to obtain a medical cannabis card is through a commercial "card mill," where you can pay less for the exact same medical card that you'd otherwise get from a specialized doctor or nurse. Here's the rub: Typically, these card mills just go through the motions of teaching you how to use cannabis safely and effectively. There are many mercenary companies that do this. They are essentially following the letter, if not the spirit, of the law, and they don't provide nearly enough helpful education or guidance, if they provide any at all. You get what you pay for. A card mill will charge you a fee of about $125, while it could cost you $200 to $450 to meet with a real cannabis doctor. At the other end of the fee spectrum, some "medical cannabis" doctors are mercenary and charge way too much for a visit. I wouldn't pay $450—that is exorbitant. It is a good idea to shop around. The fee should be in the $200 to $300 range.

If you buy cannabis infrequently and use relatively small amounts, it might not be worth the trouble and expense of getting a medical cannabis card. In this scenario, the total annual cost for cannabis products wouldn't be that high. The 20 percent that you would save from taxes and new patient specials wouldn't be significant enough to offset the yearly cost and trouble of getting a medical cannabis card.

One must renew one's medical cannabis card annually. As a physician in Massachusetts, I am allowed to renew it for two years if a patient is legally disabled. Depending on which state you live in, it is worth asking your doctor if you qualify for a longer certification period. Some doctors certify their patients for a shorter period than allowed—maybe three to six months—to extract more fees. Then they make their patients come back and pay another fee, to get the card renewed. Don't put up with a doctor who only certifies you for a very limited period, unless it is legally stipulated. In Massachusetts, for example, we are allowed to certify people for a whole year, so it is suspicious when doctors certify patients for only six months and then charge them for certification once again. Although double charging is not usually medically necessary, it could make sense in rare cases where there is a legitimate need for more frequent, complex follow-up. The laws vary from state to state, and some may specify that a patient can visit a doctor more often than once a year. Of course, medical follow-up is essential. In my practice, I often do that with patients via email and clinical direct messaging through our hospital/patient computer system—free of charge.

Always bring your medical marijuana card to the dispensary with you. Remember that some dispensaries are "medical" and will accept your card. Others are "medical and recreational" and will also accept your card. If it just a "recreational" dispensary, you can still buy marijuana, as a legal adult, but you won't get any of the discounts and other perks that come with a medical marijuana card. At a recreational store you will be treated as a recreational customer—and you will need to pay taxes.

## ADDITIONAL POINTS ABOUT DISPENSARIES

There are a few more things that are helpful to know before you visit a dispensary. For example, many dispensaries offer senior discounts, but when you go, remember to bring identification. You will need it, not only to purchase cannabis products but also to get into the dispensary itself. If you are too disabled to go to a dispensary by yourself, you can either designate a caregiver to shop for you, or you can take advantage of home delivery services, which are now available in many places.

### Senior Discounts

Many medical dispensaries offer senior discounts. At medical dispensaries, senior discounts are added to benefits that you're already getting with your medical card. Some recreational dispensaries also offer senior discounts. For example, some dispensaries in Massachusetts give a 10 percent discount to people who are sixty-five and older.

### Identification

As previously mentioned, always take identification (e.g., a valid, government-issued photo ID such as driver's license) to any dispensary, whether it's recreational or medical. You won't get in or purchase anything without it. Take your medical cannabis card as well, if you have one, if it's required in your state.

## Payment

You must take cash or a bank card to all dispensaries, medical or otherwise. Most dispensaries are allowed to accept bank cards but not credit cards.

## Designating a Caregiver

If you are too weak or frail to go to a medical dispensary on your own, or if you are homebound, most medical marijuana states will allow you to designate a caregiver to go to the dispensary on your behalf. Your caregiver is allowed to purchase cannabis products for you under the auspices of your medical marijuana card. Unfortunately, many medical marijuana states do not allow patients to bring anyone else with them into a medical dispensary, so you can't usually go in with your caregiver. If it is a recreational dispensary, anyone over the age of twenty-one can go in with you, but you can't use your medical card and won't be eligible for tax breaks or other benefits of a medical marijuana card.

## Delivery Services

An increasing number of dispensaries are offering delivery services for medical patients. Please check your state regulations to see which ones apply to you. Home deliveries can be another convenient option for patients who have trouble getting to a dispensary.

## Reciprocity

Many states have reciprocity with other states for medical cards. For example, if my medical marijuana card was issued to me in Massachusetts, I can use it in Maine to get into medical dispensaries there. A person with a medical marijuana card from Maine can likewise use it at dispensaries in Massachusetts. Cannabis in

Maine is about half as expensive as it is in Massachusetts, so many people drive there to shop. If you use a substantial amount of cannabis products, it may be worth evaluating where it is most economical to buy it.

Make sure that the state you are going to for bargain-hunting has good regulation of their cannabis products. Less stringent regulation may be one reason the prices are so much lower. If the product is worse, it might not be worth purchasing it—even if it costs less. If you are shopping for cannabis in a different state, you can't legally fly with it (see page 167 for more information) and you should be aware that it is illegal to cross state borders with cannabis, although this is usually somewhat of a technicality as most states generally don't police their borders for this, except possibly in some conservative Southern states.

## LEGAL AND OTHER CONSIDERATIONS

Be extremely careful not to run afoul of local or federal laws concerning cannabis. Cannabis is still completely illegal in some states and in other states it is legal only for medical purposes. The legality of cannabis is constantly evolving. We are generally heading in the right direction, but there are still eleven states where medical cannabis isn't legal. However, some of those states have provisions for CBD and super-low THC products. It is critical to know and follow the laws of your state and to check the laws of any other state you might be traveling to in order to minimize the chances of getting into legal trouble. This is your responsibility. You must be particularly careful when traveling with cannabis, and it is not recommended that you fly with it, even between two legal states. Do not ever travel internationally with cannabis.

## What Are the Qualifying Conditions by State for Medical Marijuana?

Regulations that specify which conditions can be certified with a medical marijuana card differ from state to state. Some are very liberal on this matter and others are quite conservative. The list is constantly changing so you might have to look it up to see what is allowed in your state. Of course, if you are in a state that has legal recreational dispensaries, you can buy cannabis for any purpose whatsoever, and even use it medically for any condition, as many people do. That would be a good workaround if your medical condition has not been approved as a "qualifying condition." Incidentally, chronic pain and insomnia are qualifying conditions in all states, whereas more specific diagnoses, like female orgasmic disorder, are recognized in some states but not in others.

## Travel

It is not legal to cross any state border if you are in possession of cannabis, due to federal illegality, as state borders are under federal control. Although that may be true, it poses only a hypothetical risk, if, say, you are driving between two contiguous legal states, such as New York and New Jersey. On the other hand, if you are driving through a state like Idaho to get from Colorado to Oregon (both legal states), you could get into trouble if cannabis is found in your possession, because it is illegal in Idaho. In a situation like that one, you must use caution. If you have cannabis in the trunk of your car, which is the safest place to store it while traveling, by the way, and if you aren't speeding or driving erratically, it's unlikely you'd be pulled over.

In the Northeast, on the West Coast, or in any other state where it is legal, police rarely care about simple cannabis possession—if you aren't doing anything wrong. It is likely to be somewhat more of a problem in conservative states, where, in some places, cannabis isn't legal yet. And there is still a tremendous amount of racial discrimination in the application of cannabis policy. Black Americans and white Americans use cannabis at the same rate, yet Black consumers are arrested for it nearly four times as often.[2] They are much more likely to be pulled over in the first place, and more likely to be searched—and criminal penalties are more severe. This is an ugly fact about our cannabis policy—naked racism, which has been exceedingly difficult to extinguish.

It is advisable not to fly domestically with cannabis because the feds, specifically the FAA (Federal Aviation Administration), regulate the transportation of illegal substances like cannabis. Certainly, never travel with anything obvious, like a pipe or a vaporizer, because it's just asking for trouble. It is unfair and counterproductive that people can't freely and legally travel with cannabinoid medicine. Restrictions often make it so that people don't have access to their medicine while traveling, and many suffer immensely as a result. Nonetheless, it is important to be aware that flying with cannabis is illegal and you could get into trouble if you don't follow the law, unreasonable as it may be. Fly with cannabis at your own risk.

Taking cannabis over international borders is even riskier. If you are driving from one country where it is legal (e.g., Canada) back to a part of the United States where it is legal (e.g., Vermont, just over the border), this is still considered an illegal act and border police could give you a hard time for it. In fact, people have even been arrested for driving from one country to another with cannabis, although it is not an enforcement priority. It is best not to travel to any other country with cannabis. Just go into a store and buy it in Canada if you need it, but don't travel with it. If you decide you need to take cannabis with you, as you travel, be extremely cautious. Understand that you are assuming a risk. Do not, under any circumstances, take it to a country that has zero tolerance, such as Russia or Saudi Arabia. You could end up in prison for a long time.

Restrictions on travel place a burden on medical cannabis users who depend on it. This is particularly true of people who divide their time between two places during the year. An example of this might be snowbirds—Northerners who spend their winters in Florida to escape cold weather in the north. Medical and recreational weed is legal in Boston. But—what will they do when they're in Florida for four months? In Florida, there is an entirely different medical system, without reciprocity, and no recreational cannabis. Are people supposed to fly with it and hope they don't get caught? Drive with it and hope they don't get caught? Pay for a separate medical cannabis doctor in Florida so they can buy it there legally? This is all quite a logistical headache: It denies patients their medication and it forces them to decide whether to break the law, spend more money, or do without.

## Hospital Etiquette

One aspect of medical cannabis that remains awkward is that patients aren't welcome to use it in the hospital. This is the case because hospitals derive a large part of their funding from the federal government. Given that cannabis remains illegal on a federal level, hospitals are worried that if they encourage, or even allow, cannabis use, their funding will be in jeopardy. The last thing hospital security guards want to do is harass medical cannabis patients or, worse, rip it out of the hands of suffering or dying patients. I have spoken in detail on this issue with hospital security personnel and it puts them in an impossible bind.

On the other hand, patients who are deriving benefit from using medical cannabis on a daily basis do not wish to stop using it because of outdated and overly restrictive laws. They don't want to physically withdraw from cannabis while they're in the hospital. It is already difficult enough to eat and sleep in a hospital, so who needs to experience cannabis withdrawal, which makes eating and sleeping all the more difficult? Their preference is to continue to use cannabis as a complement to the mainstream pharmaceuticals they are given in the hospital, such as opioids. In fact, they could even reduce their use of opioids with medical cannabis. Ideally, the use of mainstream pharmaceuticals and cannabis should be integrated into hospital-based care. Prohibition results in a lot of sneaking around, confiscation, occasional arrests, and many missed opportunities for communication between doctors and patients.

Short of full federal legalization, patients might do two things as a compromise. For one, they can be discreet about their use of medical cannabis in the hospital. Obviously, as an extreme example, it would be unwise and hugely inconsiderate to light up a joint and fumigate an entire wing of a nonsmoking hospital. Patients shouldn't use vapes or do anything that makes other patients or staff uncomfortable. Instead, they could, hypothetically, take a discreet puff from their vaporizer in a permitted smoking area for cigarette smokers, if they aren't too ill or debilitated to get to it. Alternatively, they could quietly use some unmarked gummies that they might have brought in and that no one would notice. That is, in fact, what a lot of patients do. However, it is much safer to stop all cannabis use a day or two before surgery, or any other procedure—if not earlier.

While they're in the hospital, it is of utmost importance that patients communicate with their doctors and nurses about their use of medical cannabis, even though it may be awkward at times, to avoid unwanted medication interactions or anesthesia requirements. There is only a very small chance that your medical team would alert security, as their first obligation is to you. Most doctors and nurses probably wouldn't be averse to reasonable cannabis use if it helps their patients.

## Driving and Adult Responsibilities

If you are using medical cannabis, make sure that someone else is the designated driver. The use of cannabis, especially in higher doses, can increase your odds of a car accident when you are under the influence (see chapter 5). It is also a good idea to make sure that you aren't in charge of too many major adult responsibilities while using cannabis, especially when you are just getting used to it, as cannabis can temporarily impair your functioning. The last thing you want is to be called to deal with a crisis when you have just eaten a gummy and are waiting for it to take effect. This is also true of many other impairing pain medications, such as opioids, benzodiazepines, muscle relaxants, some of the antidepressants, and sedatives.

## Finding a Doctor Who Is Knowledgeable About Cannabis

As mentioned, some doctors know a helpful amount about the medicinal use of cannabis, whereas others are still suffering from a lack of practical education on this matter. Regardless of where they stand on cannabis, it is important to have open conversations with your doctor. Start with your primary care physician. The majority of primary care physicians are supportive of medical cannabis. Most oncologists are supportive of cannabis as well, along with an increasing number of pain and addiction doctors and orthopedists.

Keep in mind that doctors can't prescribe cannabis, because it is not an FDA-approved drug. However, they can recommend it, make helpful suggestions, and then provide you with a medical card.

## Affordability

Cannabis costs are not reimbursed by health insurance companies in the United States. Depending on how much cannabis you use, it can become quite expensive. Gummies can cost a dollar or two, and if you use three a day, that comes to about $1,500 per year. Prescription cannabis medications (e.g., Marinol, Epidiolex, nabilone) are sometimes covered by insurance, but they are infrequently prescribed, and some patients don't find them to be as effective as cannabis itself.

I have successfully transitioned patients from taking Percocet and Valium—two extremely addictive and dangerous medications—to using cannabis instead, but there was literally a price to pay. My patients were doing better with medical marijuana than they had been with the use of pharmaceuticals—they had less grogginess, itchiness, and constipation, and felt that their quality of life was improved on cannabis—but as one of them told me, "On MassHealth, Percocet and Valium are costing me one dollar a month and I'm paying $150 a month for cannabis—I have to go back to the pills." That outcome is a loss for all parties involved, including the shortsighted health insurance company, which now has to pay for all those pills again.

It can be very difficult for people with a low or fixed income—veterans and retirees, for example—to afford medical cannabis. Insurance companies ought to pay for medical cannabis; they are making a killing on all the medications and treatments that patients don't need because they are using medical cannabis instead. This will eventually be fixed, but, for now, you will have to pay for cannabis on your own. Thankfully, some dispensaries have special benefits for veterans and most have senior discounts—and some states that have legalized cannabis now have provisions for growing your own, which makes consumption a lot less expensive. In Massachusetts, for example, you are allowed to have six plants per adult, per home, as long as the plants can't be seen from the street without binoculars.

## Monitoring

Ideally, anyone who has just started using medical cannabis should be monitored as carefully as any other patient who is taking a new medication. The intensity of monitoring depends somewhat on the patient. If their condition is complicated, or they are new to medical cannabis, they may need to be seen in follow-up, or at least touch base with their health care provider, within one to six months, if not within a few weeks after starting to use it. They should be encouraged to freely communicate with their health care team if they have any questions or concerns.

Any follow-up should involve appropriate monitoring for efficacy. If it's needed, a clinician can recommend changes in dosage, suggest different consumption methods or plant varieties, and monitor side effects. There is much to monitor when a patient begins treatment with medical cannabis. For example, one must be aware of potential problems with addiction (see chapter 6) or, perhaps, adverse interactions of other medications with cannabis. And of course, careful monitoring helps health care providers determine when cannabis isn't working effectively and needs to be discontinued. Some state medical registries use validated questionnaires and quality of life assessments, which allows them to track different objective measures, such as improvements in symptoms and function, as well as side effects.

## OTHER PRACTICALITIES OF CANNABIS TO CONSIDER

There are a variety of other practicalities involved in purchasing and using cannabis. These include issues such as: What are the actual effects of cannabis? What does it feel like to be high? What do you do if cannabis gives you the munchies (i.e., makes food taste unreasonably good so it is difficult to stop eating it)? What consumption products can you make at home with cannabis? What are the implications for exercise? How do we cope with any lingering stigma associated with cannabis use? How do you safely store cannabis? These questions and more are covered here.

### What Is It Like to Be High?

The experience of being high differs from person to person, but it usually results in a relaxed state of calm euphoria. Time slows down and you feel grounded in the present moment. All your senses are heightened. Vision is more vivid, and colors seem magnified, which is why some people use cannabis outdoors, to walk in the woods, where everything seems even prettier. Everything tastes better, too. That's why people often like to consume cannabis before meals or at dinner parties. The intensity and appreciation of sounds is also magnified, which is why people enjoy listening to music or seeing live shows when under the influence. Physical sensations are also enhanced, which is why many enjoy it before massages or physical intimacy with their partners. Creative insights might flit through your mind, and activities such as going to an art museum could be inspiring.

Some people feel disoriented when they're high, especially at first, until they get used to it. Much of that feeling is dose related. If you take an appropriate dose, however, you can set yourself up for a more pleasurable experience. Taking too high a dose can range from unpleasant to miserable, so it is critical to be cautious about the dose you take. Some people never get used to the high or just don't like it at all. Typically, they use only CBD.

Being high can also complement the painkilling effects of cannabis by impacting the part of our brain that interprets pain as an unpleasant sensation. In other words, people can still feel pain but not be particularly bothered by it. That distraction from pain can make it more likely for people to participate in pleasurable and meaningful activities.

## The Munchies

As depicted in popular media, cannabis can give you the munchies, because it makes everything taste better—and also makes you feel hungrier than usual. This is why cannabis is helpful for patients with cancer, anorexia of aging (an age-related reduction of appetite and food intake), HIV, long Covid, and other conditions that make consuming enough calories and gaining weight so difficult. The munchies are not particularly helpful, though, for people who are on diets and trying to limit what they eat.

Ironically, chronic cannabis users weigh less than the general population and tend to have a lower BMI (body mass index). One would think that on average, they would be portlier because they enjoy eating so much. The "why" of that phenomenon is not well understood, but it might be because cannabis users are more physically active. Or, it could have something to do with the ways in which cannabis tickles our endocannabinoid receptors and affects our metabolism.

The best way to deal with the munchies, for the majority of people who are trying to lose weight, is to be mindful about eating and get plenty of exercise. Avoid fast food and junk food as much as you can. Getting high is not a valid reason for breaking the diet you've worked so hard to maintain. If there are only healthy snacks at home, you'll limit how much damage you can do to your calorie count when you start cannabis induced grazing. Grapes, carrots, or apples, for example, taste wonderful under the influence of cannabis and aren't particularly fattening. Some experts say, "just don't start eating" but that can be difficult. If you are going to eat, make sure you have access to nutritious, low-calorie snacks.

## Exercise While on Cannabis

Drug war–era myths about cannabis users stereotypically portrayed them as lazy and unlikely to exercise or even move off the sofa. Supposedly they have "amotivational syndrome," which most experts now recognize is completely unfounded. Do cannabis users exercise more or less than people who abstain? The data is contradictory. According to one study, "Marijuana users are equal to or more likely to exercise than non-users."[3] With mindful planning, you can incorporate exercise into your cannabis use, or cannabis into your exercise, which many people find rewarding. Cannabis can improve focus, motivation, and mindfulness during exercise. Of course, you don't want to consume cannabis and then drive to your gym or yoga class, so make sure you go with a designated driver or use a ride service. Another caveat is that it is best to use machinery—such as weight machines or treadmills—with caution, as your balance may be affected.

## Things You Can Make with Cannabis

You can make a wide variety of things to eat from cannabis flower. Most commonly, people make cannabis butter or brownies. You can also easily purchase various devices, such as the

MagicalButter Machine, that make it easy to make infused foodstuffs, like ketchup and salad dressing, as well as basic tinctures. At dispensaries you can buy all kinds of infused food products like honey, chocolate, hot sauce, and pizza sauce. As mentioned previously, I don't recommend these products, however, because it is all too easy to overconsume THC—and difficult to track your dosage—if they are part of a meal. Also, having these products around the house is a recipe for disaster, if little kids or other people who shouldn't or don't want to use cannabis accidentally consume it.

#### *Brownies*

Here are a few pointers for making (and eating) marijuana brownies—a pastime that I have partaken in many times: Stir the batter thoroughly, so that all the brownies have the same concentration of THC. This is critical to ensure adequate dosing and prevent overconsumption. It doesn't help if some brownies are ten times stronger than the others because the cannabis hasn't been evenly distributed. Also, don't freely eat the brownie mix! It is highly psychoactive, and you can get way too high or start vomiting ("greening out") if you eat too much batter.

#### *Infused Dinners*

"Infused dinners" are popular new social events where a chef makes a multicourse, often gourmet, dinner using various amounts of cannabis in the food. The chefs at the dinners I have attended use only as much cannabis as each guest would like. The options include none, if you wish to enjoy the dinner and the company but cannabis doesn't sit well with you; a low dose (5–10 milligrams) over the entire dinner; a medium dose (10–15 milligrams); or a high dose (20–25 milligrams). You have control over this and must be careful not to consume too much. Infused meals are long, and the cannabis you eat is consumed slowly, over about four hours. People often smoke cannabis at these dinners between courses, so in addition to the cannabis eaten via food, you must pay very close attention to how much cannabis you are smoking (or secondhand smoke you are inhaling). Do not drive home after these events.

### Social Consumption Sites

Social consumption sites are becoming legal in a few states. California is leading the way, with Massachusetts soon to follow. In other states, these sites are more "underground," as they aren't quite legal. Going to a social consumption site is analogous to going to a bar. The idea is that you can order or use cannabis products openly at the site. Cannabis beverages might be available, and you are allowed to freely smoke cannabis. If you go to a social consumption site, make sure you have a designated driver or a ride service to get back home, and be careful to not overconsume.

### Changing Opinions About Cannabis Use

As you might expect, opinions on the subject of cannabis use vary widely among families. Fortunately, attitudes are changing for the better. Currently about 90 percent of Americans believe that people should have legal access to medical marijuana. Many of my older patients were first encouraged to use medical cannabis by their kids who were sick of seeing their parents suffer. With other families in my practice, it was the kids who were utterly shocked to see grandma toking up.

There is still a lot of stigma and misinformation floating around among older patients from the war on drugs, as evidenced in a 2024 study:

> Perceived stigma was evident in many participants' descriptions of their perceptions of cannabis in the past and present, and influenced how they accessed and consumed cannabis and their comfort in discussing its use with their health care providers. A culture shift needs to occur among health care providers so that they are educated about cannabis and willing to discuss the possibilities of medicinal cannabis consumption with older adults. Otherwise, older adults may seek advice from recreational or other non-medical sources.[4]

All of us need to move beyond the stigma of using cannabis, as it harms patients and stymies communication within families and with health care providers.

## The Fine Line Between Medical and Recreational Cannabis

The ongoing process of re-legalizing cannabis has resulted in an overstated distinction between medical use and recreational use. Since in most states there was more public sympathy for medical use, it was legalized first. This dichotomy has given rise to the belief that medical and recreational cannabis are separate and different entities, when, in fact, there is considerable overlap between medical and recreational cannabis use. Studies have consistently shown that many medical patients also frequently use cannabis recreationally. Patients don't always differentiate between the two categories. With cannabis, you might have more social enjoyment and also better pain control—it isn't always an either-or situation. Other studies have shown that people who buy cannabis in recreational shops often use it for pain, anxiety, and insomnia, which are obviously medical uses. Even if you are a medical patient, it can be easier to just go into a recreational store, in one of the twenty-five states that have legalized recreational cannabis, and buy cannabis without the expense and hassle of obtaining a medical card.

Certainly, there are times when cannabis use is purely recreational. An example of this would be the time I smoked a joint with my cousins before seeing the Who perform at Fenway Park, under a full moon. That was a great use of recreational cannabis!—not a medical one—unless you define "medical" so broadly as to include just having fun. On the other hand, a dying cancer patient isn't likely to use cannabis recreationally. That would be pure medical use. In any case, and in most cases, medical and recreational patients consume the exact same marijuana.

## Keep Original Packaging on Cannabis Products

For your safety and everyone else's, store medicinal cannabis in a private, secure place. In fact, you might consider locking it up wherever you store narcotics, benzodiazepines, and other addictive or dangerous medicines. It is critical to keep cannabis out of sight of children and pets. Don't forget—teens tend to snoop around and go through their parents' private belongings, so definitely factor that in.

If you take a cannabis product out of its original packaging, it is an open invitation for someone else to accidentally consume it. After all, how would they know it isn't a regular chocolate bar? I strongly advise keeping products in their original packaging, especially half-eaten chocolate bars. Do not leave an unmarked portion in the fridge—it never ends well. If you have mangled the label you can always create your own. My dad used to keep brownies in his freezer that he taped closed with gigantic labels that warned "DO NOT EAT." (Of course, as teenagers, we took this as an invitation, but that is a different story.)

## How to Get Involved in the Legalization Movement

If you, or members of your family, personally benefit from medical cannabis, but don't live in a legal state—or if you just think it should be legally available to sick patients—you can help work toward full legalization. Every state that isn't fully legal yet has a local legalization movement and a local chapter of NORML (National Organization for the Reform of Marijuana Laws) that is working to alleviate this problem. Local chapters of national groups like NORML and MPP (Marijuana Policy Project) are highly effective. One of my favorite groups is the Last Prisoner Project, which is dedicated to freeing people who have been jailed for cannabis offenses. There are also a lot of other local groups, including veterans' organizations, that are working on these issues—and you can easily find them on the internet.

## Fearmongering Among Medical Professionals

In my opinion, certain members of the medical community are determined to magnify the harms of cannabis. Usually, they are doctors who have never treated patients with cannabis for any medical purpose. Most haven't even tried it themselves and are thus more susceptible to the moral panic that was created during the war on drugs. Doctors are often caught in a bubble of selective information in the same way that cannabis enthusiasts can be caught in a bubble of only positive information. For an accurate description of actual harms, please see my more comprehensive book, *Seeing Through the Smoke: A Cannabis Specialist Untangles the Truth About Marijuana.*[5]

Although everyone is entitled to their own opinion, it is unhelpful when doctors are blanketly opposed to any use of medical cannabis. Patients use it anyway and just clam up when they're around their physicians if they feel they'll be criticized and judged. This unhelpful attitude ruins communication between doctors and patients and perpetuates outdated misconceptions about cannabis. If your doctor is not helpful, you may need to pay for a consultation with a medical cannabis specialist.

### How to Talk to Doctors About Using Cannabis

If you're using cannabis, my best advice is to proactively bring up the subject with your doctors, and to be open and honest with them. They are professionals who can find a way to deal with it, regardless of their personal opinions or reservations. If using cannabis to relieve your symptoms is going well, your doctor should be happy that you are finding relief and be willing to help you in this process. They should also be engaged in tracking any harms or benefits that come from cannabis use—including potential addiction. Humans have used cannabis for five thousand years to treat medical problems and there is no reason for anyone to be ashamed of using it.

CHAPTER 7

# What Role Does CBD Play in Addressing Health Issues as We Age?

CBD is the most abundant nonintoxicating cannabinoid in cannabis. Its use is incredibly common in the United States. According to the Association of American Medical Colleges, "64 percent of US adults reported trying a CBD product—and nearly half of them did so at a doctor's suggestion."[1] People claim all kinds of benefits, ranging from the legitimate to the preposterously exaggerated. The strength of the data supporting various purported benefits of CBD varies widely. CBD is legal in most of the fifty United States, although laws can vary, are subject to change, and need to be checked.

Clinically, CBD is "low-hanging fruit" compared with cannabis, as it has fewer side effects and toxicities and is not psychoactive. CBD doesn't get you high or stoned and as such, it can be a lot easier to dose during the daytime or if you need to drive or work. CBD is not addictive and isn't considered to be particularly impairing, beyond perhaps some mild sleepiness. It often makes sense to start with CBD first, before cannabis, to alleviate symptoms, especially for older adults, who are more prone to the side effects of cannabis in general. It is difficult to find a physician who is against the use of CBD.

Doctors often begin treating older patients just with CBD, especially for chronic pain, anxiety, or insomnia. CBD in some cases is not as clinically effective as THC, or a combination of CBD and THC, so eventually some THC might need to be added to augment the effect of the CBD. There is also evidence suggesting that CBD can help mitigate some of the side effects of THC, such as short-term memory impairment and anxiety—for example if the dose of THC is too high.

Seniors are using CBD quite a bit. According to a recent study:

> CBD use is common, more so than cannabis, especially in the 65+ age group, and positively correlated with both medical and nonmedical cannabis use. . . . In the 50–64 age group, 18.3 percent and 18.0 percent reported past-year CBD and cannabis, respectively, use. In the 65+ age group, the percentages were 14.3 percent and 8.0 percent.[2]

In another study, 8 percent of those over the age of sixty-five used CBD, mostly for pain (40 percent), anxiety (20 percent), insomnia (11 percent), and arthritis (8 percent).[3]

I often advocate for starting just with CBD, unless a patient is suffering from one of the conditions that THC is uniquely qualified for, such as chemotherapy-induced nausea and vomiting, migraine, anorexia, or severe chronic pain.

In 2021, a group of physicians came up with some suggestions for dosing CBD and medical cannabis. For older patients, especially those who are new to cannabis, they recommend a more conservative initiation into cannabinoid medicine. Specifically, they recommend starting at a very low dose of CBD, at 5–10 milligrams, going up by 5–10 milligrams every several days. Once you reach a dose of 40 milligrams of CBD per day, they suggest adding a small amount (just 1 milligram) of THC.[4]

Here is a chart of their recommendations:

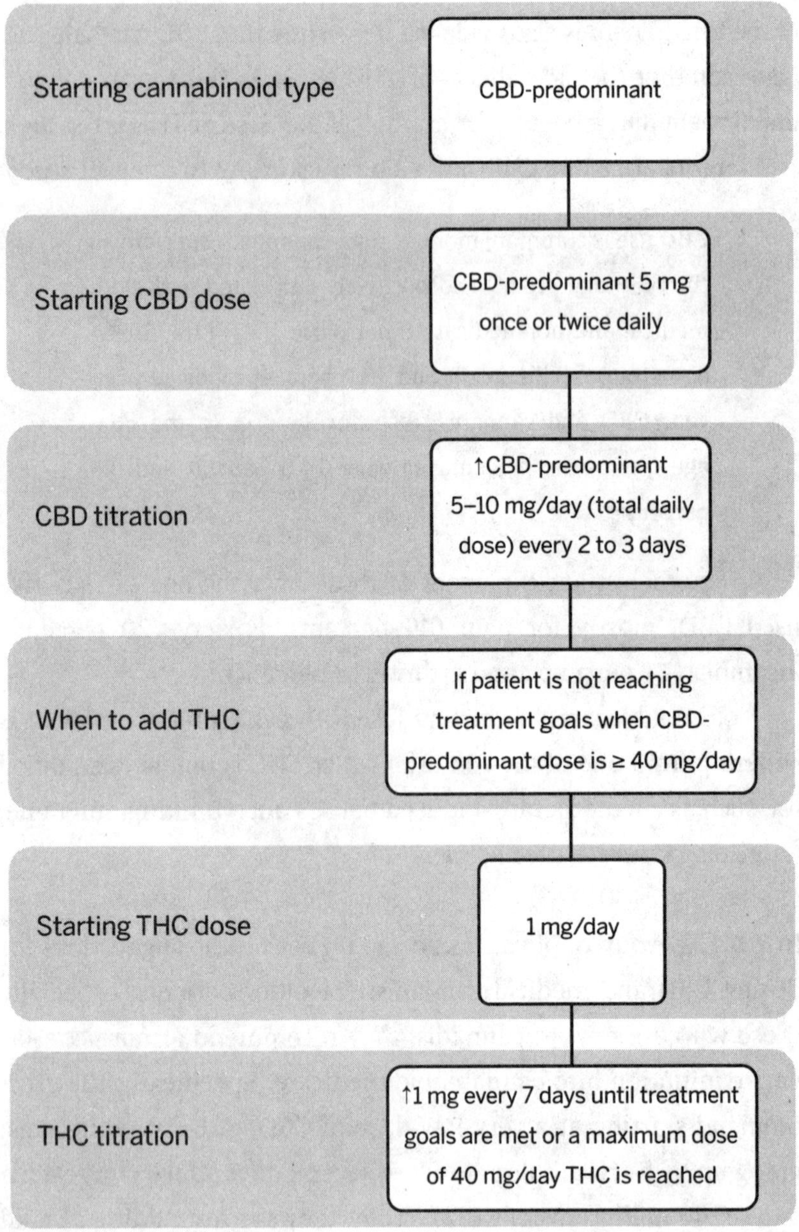


*Source: Bhaskar, A. et al. "Consensus Recommendations on Dosing and Administration of Medical Cannabis to Treat Chronic Pain," Journal of Cannabis Research, Springer Nature, 2021 (see note 4 for chapter 7 on page 248).*

Generally, I agree with the physicians' recommendations, although I would likely start with a higher dose of CBD than just 5 milligrams. One would need a larger dose than that to derive a therapeutic benefit. I would start in the 10–25 milligram range, and I might go up higher than 40 milligrams, which is a relatively small dose, before switching to THC. With older patients, we think it best to start conservatively to avoid side effects and drug interactions, but we still need to give an adequate therapeutic dose.

Optimal dosing of CBD for older patients hasn't been studied, so we are largely extrapolating from studies involving younger patients. However, optimal dosing hasn't been well studied in that group, either. Older patients might need lower doses of CBD because their liver and kidneys don't work as well as those of younger patients. Many studies show that a helpful dose of CBD to alleviate symptoms should be in the hundreds of milligrams. For example, one study, which did not focus specifically on older people, found that "therapeutic benefits of CBD became more clearly evident at doses greater than or equal to 300 mg. Increased dosing from 60 to 400 mg/day did not appear to be associated with an increased frequency of adverse effects."[5]

Another issue related to dosing is that only about 10 percent of CBD (from 6–18 percent) is absorbed when it is taken orally. In other words, if you are taking a 30-milligram gummy, and absorbing 10 percent of the CBD, you might be getting about 3 milligrams, which is a homeopathic dose. This dose certainly wouldn't accomplish anything much, except cost you money. Even if you absorbed the entire 30 milligram dose, it might not be a high enough dose to have any effect. Tinctures placed under your tongue are more effective because they are absorbed directly into your bloodstream (see pages 34–37).

CBD can become expensive at therapeutic doses, too, especially in the range of hundreds of milligrams. Insurance doesn't cover CBD, and 30 milligram gummies typically cost a dollar or two. This means that, if you took CBD daily, you would spend hundreds to thousands of dollars per year, none of which would be reimbursed. The CBD-based drug Epidiolex, which is used to treat seizure disorders, including childhood epilepsy, is covered by insurance, but it has a very narrow indication, i.e., it can only be used for a limited set of conditions—in this case, childhood epilepsy.

The quality of commercial CBD can be shockingly poor, as no one is regulating the industry. Be careful to obtain CBD from a reputable, reliable source. Study after study has shown that many of CBD products found in stores, smoke shops, and online are wildly mislabeled. Some of them, such as CBD beverages, didn't contain any CBD at all, while others had more CBD in the contents than their labels claimed. Still other products were found to contain significant amounts of THC, which could be disastrous if you weren't expecting anything other than CBD in the product you purchased and consumed—especially if you were driving home from the store. The industry truly needs an adult in the room to regulate it but so far the US government has declined to do so, even though CBD is a multibillion-dollar industry.

The best way to navigate the poor quality of commercial CBD is to make sure that a COA (Certificate of Analysis) label is included with any CBD you purchase. This label demonstrates that the vendor or manufacturer has subjected its samples to independent laboratory testing. These analyses are reasonably accurate, as the labs are usually confirmed and accredited. However, some labs are substandard, and some companies even stoop to lab shopping, where they engage various labs to test their products, and then advertise the "best" results. Whatever you do, don't purchase CBD in a gas station or smoke shop. In all likelihood it won't be CBD, and it could even be something dangerous. Make sure you buy CBD from a company that provides independent laboratory testing.

As mentioned in chapter 5, it's important to be very careful with CBD and potential drug interactions. That's because, just like grapefruit juice, CBD can compete with other substances for the use of your liver enzymes and make them less available to remove other medications from the blood. That being the case, CBD can elevate the level of other drugs in your body, which are metabolized more slowly, and can impact medications that need to stay within a narrow therapeutic range, such as blood thinners, antiepileptics, and immunosuppressants. For example, one study showed that the level of tacrolimus, an immunosuppressant, can go up 4.2 times with the co-administration of CBD, and thus requires both a dosage reduction and close clinical monitoring.[6] The study demonstrates the need to watch the levels of other drugs when taking CBD and shows why it is important to discuss your CBD usage with all your doctors.

Although it happens rarely, a person's liver can become inflamed when using CBD. Inflammation is often seen at very high doses of CBD, however, and with the co-administration of other drugs, such as antiepileptics (e.g., valproic acid). When you start using CBD, liver tests should be monitored, particularly at high doses of CBD, or if CBD is being taken with certain other medications. Liver tests should be reviewed, periodically, during regular primary care or specialty visits.

## MAIN USES OF CBD

Millions of patients are now using CBD, but what are they using it for? The list of potential indications seems to grow each year. The most established uses of CBD help to alleviate anxiety, insomnia, and chronic pain. CBD is an FDA-approved medication for certain intractable childhood epilepsy syndromes, and there is increasing evidence that it can help with conditions as diverse as autism, addiction, and agitation in Alzheimer's patients.

A 2021 Canadian real-world study evaluated the use patterns of almost ten thousand older Canadian medical cannabis patients and showed that 83.6 percent of them used CBD-based preparations containing only or mostly CBD.

> The majority of older adults reported improvements in pain (72.7 percent), sleep (64.5 percent), and mood (52.8 percent), with 35.6 percent reporting use of a reduced dose of opioids and 19.9 percent a reduced dose of benzodiazepines. . . . Users reported improved pain, sleep, and mood symptoms at follow-up after cannabis use.[7]

The use of fewer opioids and benzos will likely translate into fewer lives lost. CBD is not addictive; it is less toxic than opioids or benzos; and it is virtually impossible to have an overdose.

## Anxiety

One classic study showed how effective CBD can be in stressful situations: "CBD significantly reduced anxiety, cognitive impairment and discomfort in their speech performance, and significantly decreased uncomfortable arousal in their anticipatory speech. The placebo group presented higher anxiety, cognitive impairment, discomfort, and alert levels when compared with the control group."[8]

The dose used in the study was a hefty 600 milligrams, higher than the 5–40 milligrams suggested in the dosing chart (see page 184), although one must remember to be cautious about dosing in older patients. This was a placebo-controlled study, so the researchers demonstrated that the effect was not simply due to the placebo. A second study added, "The data suggest that CBD may reduce anxiety with minimal adverse effects when compared to a placebo."[9] The authors of this study remind us that the data set they were working from could have been more complete. We are behind in studying the ways in which CBD can help alleviate anxiety in humans.

In patients with Alzheimer's disease, one small study assessed anxiety levels after patients were given a high CBD/low THC formulation and reported, "Five patients have completed the 8-week trial, and all have demonstrated a reduction in anxiety relative to baseline, with some patients also demonstrating improvements in cognition."[10]

CBD can also lower the anxiety of caregivers, as this study demonstrated: "CBD-rich oil is an effective and safe therapy for treating NPS [neuropsychiatric symptoms] in AD [Alzheimer's disease] patients, while also reducing the caregivers' distress."[11]

## Chronic Pain

Many older people use CBD to alleviate chronic pain. CBD, by itself, can often provide pain control. Sometimes, when CBD is not strong enough to control pain on its own, it is supplemented with THC. Using CBD is generally safer than using opioids or NSAIDs, both of which can be harmful. CBD will not cause an addiction or harm one's kidneys. If CBD is used with or instead other drugs (like opioids or NSAIDs), and if it lowers the number or amount of more toxic medications that you need to take, then that is a win. One study, a summation of 15 other studies, showed a 42 percent reduction of pain with the use of CBD alone. It also showed a 66 percent reduction of pain when CBD was taken with THC, thereby demonstrating that the addition of a small amount of THC can be effective.[12]

Pain and inflammation are often closely linked—for example, an inflamed joint and inflammatory nerve pain, or a pinched nerve and diabetic neuropathy. As a potent anti-inflammatory, CBD also helps treat pain by that mechanism. As a recent study found, "There is sufficient clinical and preclinical evidence of CBD in pain treatment, so CBD could be an effective and safe treatment in reducing pain due to its analgesic and anti-inflammatory properties."[13] NSAIDs also help with inflammation and reducing pain, but they are more harmful to the GI (gastrointestinal) system and the kidneys than CBD.

## Insomnia

CBD can make people sleepy, which can be an unwanted side effect, if it is taken during the day—and you wish stay alert. The level of sleepiness caused by CBD depends on the dosage and individual response. The fact that CBD makes people drowsy supports the idea that CBD can help with insomnia. According to a study, "CBD alone or with equal quantities of THC may be beneficial in alleviating the symptoms of insomnia . . . all studies reported improvement in the insomnia symptoms of at least a portion of their participants."[14]

Scientific evidence increasingly suggests that using a combination of CBD and THC is more effective for treating insomnia than is using CBD alone. Sleep is an extremely complicated phenomenon, with several stages and a complex architecture, and the ways in which CBD and other cannabinoids help regulate it requires more research. However, there is a tremendous amount of anecdotal evidence suggesting that CBD by itself helps people get a good night's sleep. It doesn't make sense that millions of people use CBD for that purpose if it doesn't do anything. If that were the case, it would only be a very expensive placebo. In fact, CBD does help you feel sleepy, and it can also help contain anticipatory insomnia—the anxiety that we have about not being able to sleep, and that makes it so difficult to fall asleep.

## OTHER USES OF CBD

As we learn more about CBD through academic research, we're discovering its effectiveness—and potential effectiveness—for a variety of conditions. For example, CBD can help alleviate some childhood epilepsy syndromes that other medications can't ameliorate, and there is some evidence that CBD can work as an antipsychotic for people with conditions such as schizophrenia. Scientists are also conducting exciting research into the potential of CBD to help treat addiction and autism.

### Epilepsy

CBD is currently an FDA-approved medicine for certain difficult-to-control childhood epilepsy syndromes, such as Dravet syndrome and LGS (Lennox-Gastaut syndrome). Epidiolex is the prescription version of CBD. The dosages that are used to treat epilepsy are higher than the doses commonly used for other indications and can run in the high hundreds to thousands of milligrams. Consequently, patients are monitored for liver enzyme elevation and drug interactions.

The benefit of using CBD to address childhood epilepsy has been conclusively proven, which is why it received FDA approval. This raises the question of whether CBD might be an important component of adult epilepsy treatments when more data is available. In one study, CBD helped adults tolerate other epilepsy medications and also resulted in those patients' having "higher quality of life and lower psychiatric symptom severity."[15] In another study of patients with treatment-resistant epilepsy "the compiled analysis showed that the patients who received cannabidiol experienced a 41 percent reduction in the total number of seizures, compared to an average reduction of 18 percent in placebo groups."[16] In other words, CBD will likely prove to be helpful for adults, not just kids, with seizure disorders, but that hasn't been definitively settled. If you have epilepsy, please consult with your neurologist before adding any CBD to your regimen.

## Antipsychotic

People can suffer from psychosis at any age. CBD has antipsychotic properties, unlike THC, which is pro-psychotic and can contribute to psychotic events (see chapter 5). One study found that "CBD, either as monotherapy or added to regular antipsychotic medication, improved symptoms in patients with schizophrenia, with particularly promising effects in the early stages of illness."[17]

CBD is actively being studied to find out if it can fit into antipsychotic medicine regimens. CBD might help mitigate some of the pro-psychotic side effects of THC in patients with psychotic disorders (who, in all likelihood, shouldn't be using THC in the first place). Due to the potentially moderating effects of CBD on THC's pro-psychotic and other properties, it is thought that cannabis strains, or types, with higher CBD are safer to use than strains that consist of pure THC.[18]

## Anti-Addictive

Both animal and human studies have shown that CBD has emerging anti-addictive properties. However, this field is still a work in progress, research-wise, as we need more human studies to show that CBD is truly effective. Addiction is extremely complicated. It works by co-opting a person's brain function and can also be compounded by learning unhelpful behavioral patterns. It takes a while to figure out how new drug treatments might work and be helpful.

However, some human as well as animal data indicates that CBD can help with addiction to cigarettes, stimulants, alcohol, cannabis, and opioids. Specifically, CBD might help with the cues and cravings that cause many people to use and relapse. CBD can also cause people who are addicted to use fewer drugs, short of complete recovery. One study showed that "a single 800-mg oral dose of cannabidiol reduced the salience and pleasantness of cigarette cues, compared with a placebo, after overnight cigarette abstinence in dependent smokers."[19]

With addiction, "salience"—the exaggerated importance or attention a user places on a drug—and "cues" (for example, you see a syringe or a bottle of booze and have the overwhelming urge to use) are huge drivers of drug use, regardless of the drug involved. If CBD can help with this component of addiction, it could go a long way toward helping to alleviate addictive disorders.

In a different study, researchers assessed whether CBD could reduce cue-induced cravings in patients with heroin use disorder who were newly abstinent. The scientists gave their test subjects either 400 or 800 milligrams of CBD once daily for three consecutive days and demonstrated that, in both groups, CBD "significantly reduced both craving and anxiety induced by the presentation of salient drug cues compared with neutral cues." This effect lasted for seven days, even though patients were given CBD for only three days. There was also objective proof of a benefit in that CBD lessened the stress response, which was measured by cortisol levels and heart rate: "CBD reduced the drug cue–induced physiological measures of heart rate and salivary cortisol levels." The CBD was well tolerated.[20]

## Dermatological Concerns

One interesting study showed that the use of CBD and CBG (cannabigerol—a minor cannabinoid) was effective in reducing itching and improving the quality of life of patients who had atopic dermatitis, an inflammatory skin condition. In some cases it led to a remission.[21]

There are also claims that CBD can be helpful in preventing wrinkles, although this has not been definitively established. (For more information about skin conditions, see pages 99–102.)

## Anti-Inflammatory/Neuroprotective

CBD is known for its anti-inflammatory and neuroprotective properties, which is why it is currently being studied in animals and humans to see if it can ameliorate the effects—and perhaps help prevent and delay the progression—of some of the cruelest diseases, such as Alzheimer's, ALS (Lou Gehrig's disease), Parkinson's, and Huntington's.

Although researchers are hopeful that CBD can effectively address various neurodegenerative disorders, it isn't ready for showtime just yet. We need more concrete evidence that CBD can be used for those purposes. In 2014, my father, Dr. Lester Grinspoon, a legendary cannabis researcher, asked the NFL to investigate whether CBD could help prevent or lessen the crippling effects of CTE (chronic traumatic encephalopathy) on players who were getting too many concussions. CTE causes early onset dementia and severe psychiatric problems. My father did not hear back from the NFL, so he sent an open letter to *VICE* magazine.[22] Years later, the NFL has started pursuing exactly the type of research my dad suggested. The organization is currently investing millions of dollars into studying CBD's potential ability to provide neuroprotection from CTE.

## CBD DOES NOT INTERFERE WITH DAYTIME ACTIVITIES

Using, or at least starting with, just CBD has numerous advantages over using a cocktail of cannabis and THC. This is particularly true if you need to be clearheaded for daytime activities, such as driving a car or looking after your grandchildren. Although you might get a little bit sleepy from CBD, depending on the dosage and on how you react to it, it won't make you high or stoned. You certainly won't become incapacitated or nonfunctional as you might with a high dose of THC. In fact, you will likely be more functional if your pain and anxiety are under control. For many people, those considerations make a CBD-only regimen significantly more convenient than any formulation with THC.

Driving after consuming CBD is generally thought to be safe. One study stated that "acute, oral CBD treatment does not appear to induce feelings of intoxication and is unlikely to impair cognitive function or driving performance."[23] As with any new drug or medicine, however, you should not drive immediately after taking the first dose of CBD or after any change in dosage or brand, just in case it does make you sleepy, or in the very unlikely event that you have some other reaction to it, such as vomiting or diarrhea.

Many people with conditions such as chronic pain or anxiety, take only CBD during the day so that they can be functional. Then, in the early evening, when they don't have to drive and have fewer adult responsibilities, they incorporate some THC into the mix to help control their symptoms.

### Other Indications

People generally use CBD for many of the same reasons that they use whole cannabis, which were detailed in chapter 4, including to alleviate difficulties with IBS (irritable bowel syndrome), IBD (inflammatory bowel disease), cancer-related symptoms, migraine, fibromyalgia, and autism. They often start with CBD and work their way up to including more THC in their regimen. Older patients must be particularly cautious about the side effects of using CBD and THC, as well as their interactions with other medications they may be taking.

## HOW MINOR CANNABINOIDS CAN HELP

The other minor cannabinoids (first introduced in chapter 2) are molecules in the cannabis plant that interact with the endocannabinoid system, and that are increasingly thought to have beneficial health effects. They are often taken with CBD or THC for added effect. Just like CBD, most of them are largely free of intoxicating effects.

We are starting to see products such as CBN to aid sleep, CBG to help relieve pain and anxiety, and CBDA to reduce inflammation in the tinctures and edibles that are on sale, along with CBD. I give a very short description of those products below, in case you encounter them and wish to incorporate them into your regimen. Generally, they are thought to be harmless and potentially helpful. The research on many of these compounds is still in its infancy, so take claims of any health benefits with a large grain of salt. Just as with CBD, advertising and marketing claims are soaring above the evidence base and many have not been fully proven—at least not yet.

When I have muscle aches from weightlifting or swimming I use different tinctures of nonintoxicating cannabinoids. I start with CBD but also include CBDA, a stronger anti-inflammatory, or

CBG, which purportedly is good for muscle aches and inflammation. They seem to alleviate muscle aches about as well as NSAIDs. In any case, they are almost certainly less harmful than NSAIDs, which can destroy your heart, GI system, and kidneys.

The four main "minor" cannabinoids that you are likely to run across are:

1. **CBDA (Cannabidiolic acid):** This is the "acidic" version of CBD that is found in the cannabis plant. It is thought to be a much more potent anti-inflammatory than CBD, which is impressive because CBD itself is an effective anti-inflammatory. Pain and inflammation are often two sides of the same coin, which is why anti-inflammatories are thought to help with pain control.

2. **CBG (Cannabigerol):** CBG is thought to help stimulate appetite, especially among older adults with poor appetite or who need relief from anxiety, depression, the symptoms of colitis (including those of inflammatory bowel disease), or muscle aches etc. One placebo-controlled study reported that there was "a significant main effect of CBG on overall reductions in anxiety."[24] There is also growing interest in potentially using CBG to help prevent or treat neurodegenerative diseases, such as Parkinson's or MS, because of its anti-inflammatory properties. These uses are still under investigation.

3. **CBN (Cannabinol):** CBN is also known as the main component in "sleepy old cannabis." If you leave marijuana sitting around for years the THC degrades into CBN, which is thought to promote sleep. Thus, older cannabis can have more of a sleep-inducing effect than fresh cannabis. Many gummies now

contain CBN, often along with CBD and/or THC, and are being promoted for insomnia relief. CBN is also thought to be helpful for pain control, particularly if you have insomnia due to chronic pain, and to promote appetite, which can be useful for debilitated patients who are struggling to maintain their weight.

4. **CBC (Cannabichromene):** The benefits of CBC have mostly been shown in animal studies. CBC is thought to help with pain, inflammation, and depression.

Overall, CBD is an effective treatment—or an adjunct to treatment—that is relatively low risk and is being researched for its potential application to a host of conditions. As time goes on, we will have more precise information on how we can benefit from using CBD and other emerging cannabinoids.

CHAPTER 8

# Beyond the Medicinal: Lifestyle Improvements for Older Patients

Many patients have found that cannabis enhances and aids their enjoyment and engagement in life, in ways that transcend strictly medical applications. This is particularly true of elderly patients who, at times, struggle just to get through the day without too much pain, anxiety, loneliness, or boredom. They have discovered that when their symptoms have been effectively treated, it is easier to enjoy a walk, book group, Scrabble game, group outing, or Zumba class without as much misery and isolation. In short, when it is dosed at the right level, cannabis can improve many aspects of one's lifestyle and enjoyment of the day-to-day. People have enjoyed those benefits for thousands of years, but they haven't been fully explored in our society because any discourse on the subject was suppressed during the war on drugs. One might reasonably ask: how can this plant be so evil if it helps people relax, laugh, and dance? Don't all of us need more joy in our lives?

In discussing this issue, I don't want to sound as if I'm advocating for the recreational use of cannabis, although I am an advocate of *legalizing* cannabis for recreational use. No one should be arrested or penalized for using cannabis in that capacity. In chapter 5, I discussed the potential harms of cannabis, making it clear that I am not in favor of recommending cannabis to all of my patients, unless it helps more than it harms them.

In addition to discussion of cannabis's harms and medicinal benefits, any intellectually honest and helpful debate about the use of marijuana must include a conversation about why and how people are using it to improve their lives. Only by knowing the entire truth about it—the good, the bad, and the munchie—can people truly make informed decisions. It is more helpful for patients to understand why and how cannabis can be used recreationally, rather than just giving them a sanctimonious wag of the finger. In the background of this discussion, it is important to remember that there can be a very thin line between recreational and medical cannabis use.

## SEX

Let's talk about sex. There are different ways in which cannabis can help people connect or reconnect more deeply on a sexual level, at any age, assuming that they are physically healthy enough to participate in sexual activity. Cannabis can help people to relax, focus, and mindfully connect to the present moment. It intensifies sensory perceptions, especially touch. Cannabis can help people achieve orgasm and also make it more intense and satisfying. One study, quoted below, is among several that demonstrate the degree to which cannabis can help women with FOD (female orgasmic disorder; see also page 92).

> Among participants who experienced challenges in achieving orgasm, 72.8 percent reported that cannabis use before partnered sex increased orgasm frequency, 67 percent stated that it improved orgasm satisfaction, and 71 percent indicated that cannabis use made orgasm easier. The frequency of cannabis use before partnered sex correlated with increased orgasm frequency for women who experienced difficulties achieving orgasm.[1]

Under the influence of cannabis, men can enjoy more intense and satisfying orgasms as well.

In addition, cannabis can help people enjoy sex despite suffering from medical conditions or chronic pain. One study showed that cannabis suppositories, as well as the use of cannabis by more traditional means, can help women who are recovering from gynecological cancer improve their sex lives.

> Sexual function, including arousal, lubrication and orgasms, improved in the COCM [cannabis suppository] group; in addition, sexual pain was reduced in the COCM groups . . . feedback suggested that cannabis mediated the effects of mindful compassion and supported well-being, sexual self-efficacy, and quality of life.[2]

One of the most eloquent people to have written on this subject—in a very personal way—is the famous astronomer and Pulitzer Prize–winner Carl Sagan, who observed:

> Cannabis also enhances the enjoyment of sex—on the one hand it gives an exquisite sensitivity, but on the other hand it postpones orgasm: in part by distracting me with the profusion of images passing before my eyes. The actual duration of orgasm seems to lengthen greatly, but this may be the usual experience of time expansion which comes with cannabis smoking.[3]

Some people who use cannabis-infused lubricants and rubs claim that they enhance sexual pleasure in general. I don't know of any science that supports those claims, but it is difficult to see any harms involved.

## PLAYING AND LISTENING TO MUSIC

There is a solid reason why so many musicians use cannabis before playing music with each other. People joke that one of the biggest consequences of cannabis legalization is going to be an explosion in the number of new jam bands. Many truths are said in jest! Cannabis helps with musical expression, improvisation, creativity, and mindfulness. It also improves the dynamic interplay between musicians, and their ability to listen and coordinate with each other. Of course, the amount of cannabis consumed must be at the right dose—after all, if one is hallucinating or stoned to smithereens, it doesn't particularly help one's musicianship.

People frequently consume cannabis before concerts for the same reason. In my youth, I went to Grateful Dead concerts, among others, both with and without using cannabis, although, I have to say, the experience was profoundly more meaningful, textured, spiritual, nuanced, and enjoyable with cannabis. On those occasions, I was truly in the moment, perceived every note, and was able to appreciate the harmony between the different musicians. I was also able to feel at one with the crowd, which is a wonderful thing at a Grateful Dead concert. Cannabis was a huge component of the creative musical explosion of the 1960s and 1970s.

The deepening of musical appreciation can be invaluable for older patients, whether they are veteran musicians or newcomers, or just trying to enjoy a concert with friends.

## CREATING AND VIEWING ART

For more than a millennium people have used cannabis to help create art—for the simple reason that it stimulates the creative process. It allows people to have ideas that they wouldn't usually have and see patterns, and even see colors, that they wouldn't ordinarily perceive. I know many artists—painters—who take a toke or two before they start working and find that it unleashes their creative juices. Cannabis can help people connect with their inner child and recapture childlike wonder, confidence, and enthusiasm. It can also help you get into a flow state, where you're so absorbed in the moment that you lose track of any insecurities or inhibitions.

Some people also report having much more profound experiences at art galleries, viewings, or exhibitions under the influence of a modest dose of cannabis. They appreciate themes and images that ordinarily would pass them by and can delve more "three-dimensionally" into works of art. I have experienced this myself, and it is always a deep, moving experience. Going to a museum under the influence of cannabis can truly be profoundly inspirational and educational, often more so than it might be without using cannabis. Those insights often persist long after you've left the museum.

## CREATIVE WRITING

Many authors, this humble author included, use cannabis to increase the flow, creativity, depth, and humor in their writing. Some people do freewriting when stoned, and then edit their work the next day when the cannabis has worn off. Major luminaries report doing this, including my dad, Lester Grinspoon, who produced eleven books and 180 scientific papers at Harvard Medical, and Carl Sagan. The list of famous authors who use cannabis is endless. If you are suffering from writer's block, cannabis can help tremendously by kick-starting the flow of new ideas.

## NATURE

If there is one universally recognized benefit of consuming cannabis, it is the mindful enjoyment of the wonders of nature. Cannabis can be considered a mild psychedelic drug, and under its influence colors, sounds, and textures become more vivid. You can have an extremely pleasurable time just noticing the subtleties of light and staring at the blue sky and clouds. In the presence of nature, it is easier to enter a peaceful, calm state, and stop worrying about other concerns. You can feel childlike wonder again. Sounds and smells become more vivid with the crunch of fall leaves underfoot. The patterns on the bark of trees become more intricate—and you are more likely to notice complex fractal patterns. The quiet of nature can be profoundly peaceful and the whisper of the wind healing. Cannabis makes it easier to appreciate the pure splendor and raw beauty of wildlife, transforming a simple walk in the woods into a deeply spiritual experience.

## FOOD/COOKING

Cannabis is a popular guest at dinner parties because it facilitates one's sense of smell and taste, as well as conversation and bonhomie. Everything tastes better on cannabis—this is a universal truth. People find themselves improvising with spices, iterating on recipes, playing fun music, dancing around while they cook, and using the creativity that cannabis fosters to experiment with and improve their cooking. Cannabis supports laughter and conversation, and it can serve as an intellectual stimulant, leading to enhanced social connections. Cooking together can turn into a uniquely fun and meaningful activity.

Although others might enjoy a glass of red wine while cooking—there is, of course, nothing wrong with that, if it is okay with their doctor—cannabis is generally a healthier alternative. In fact, in some settings, cannabis is replacing alcohol as the social lubricant of choice, whether consumed in a gummy or as a puff of a shared joint. If you choose to smoke, try to make sure no one is sick before sharing a joint; you don't want to get sick while you're enjoying the company. Sometimes people bring small individual joints to consume with friends at a gathering. With each person using their own joint, the experience is more sanitary, if less of a shared ritual.

It is best not to combine alcohol and cannabis at the same time, as the sedating effects can be additive, and one can become more quickly impaired than if one were to use either alcohol or cannabis alone. Using both together can also increase the risk of falls and accidents, particularly if you drive home after a social event, which is not at all recommended. These days there are ride services, or you can designate a sober driver.

Marijuana can also make going out to a restaurant a much more enjoyable and stimulating experience. It can help you to become much more deeply immersed in the colors, smells, and tastes of the food, and to enjoy the lively atmosphere around you. To that end, social consumption sites, lounges where you can openly consume cannabis in a restaurant or club, are just starting to pop up in a few recreationally legal states (see page 177). I am in favor of this, as it facilitates social connection, which is a win, and it is safer than drinking. But, if you go to one of these lounges, you absolutely need a designated driver (or an Uber/Lyft) to get home safely. As discussed in chapter 5, people who have consumed cannabis can mistakenly think it is safe to drive home hours before it is actually safe to do so.

The fact that cannabis makes food taste so good can be a problem for people who are struggling to shrink or maintain their waistlines. Even if you've just eaten a large meal, there is always room for something yummier after consuming marijuana—it truly keeps you hungry and makes you crave food. The fact that everything tastes better is not particularly helpful to those of us on diets. I suspect that cannabis will prove to undermine the effects of new weight loss drugs like semaglutide (Wegovy and Ozempic) and tirzepatide (Zepbound and Mounjaro), at least somewhat. One way to do damage control is to exercise restraint at the supermarket, so that the only snacks you have at home are healthy fruits and vegetables. Fruit tastes phenomenal when you're high, and there is only so much damage you can do to your diet with apples or grapes (see page 174)..

## PHYSICAL ACTIVITIES/SPORTS

For decades, cannabis has been painted as a scary drug that causes "amotivational syndrome," an imaginary affliction that turns people into listless couch potatoes. While we know it's true that some people certainly enjoy lounging on their sofa when stoned and listening to the Grateful Dead, we also know that amotivational syndrome was a creation of the war on drugs. All things being equal, chronic cannabis users tend to be more active than nonusers—and many people find that sports, such as jogging and biking, are more engaging and fun, or at least less boring, with cannabis use (see page 175). Other people believe that cannabis can improve a workout, and there's some science to back up those claims.[4] In any case, they report more focus and a more mindful connection to the present and to their bodies.

I have found that cannabis, at the right dose, can vastly improve my coordination. For example, I remember one time when my twin brother and I got high as young adults. We were playing basketball—a game at which I am exceptionally mediocre—and after a few puffs, I literally couldn't miss a basket. This went on for about an hour. I think it was the first basketball game I'd ever won. Similarly, as a teen, I was eerily better at pinball when high—it gave me a better sense of where the ball was headed. I don't recommend that teenagers use cannabis but, when I was a teen, like most teens, I didn't care about warnings, which could have been a real problem. Our message to teenagers now is to just wait.

Cannabis, including CBD and the minor cannabinoid CBG, can also be effective for helping people recover from a workout. These substances can help with sore muscles and fatigue. A modest use of cannabis can also help older patients, who often have some degree of muscle or nerve pain, to engage with and participate more readily in appropriate physical activities. Cannabis can have a downstream effect by improving mood and sleep. It can also help get you into a positive feedback cycle. For example, if you are suffering from a painful condition such as fibromyalgia, you might have to limit some activities. If you use cannabis under those circumstances, however, you might experience some pain, but not enough to prevent you from participating in enjoyable activities, such as a walk outside. Then, being more active, and less isolated, you might feel less pain, or at least dwell on it less.

## DANCING

Dancing can be difficult for some seniors who may have developed arthritis or other physical limitations. Yet, it is one of the healthiest activities that people find most enjoyable. Cannabis can help. You don't have to be a dancing master like John Travolta in *Saturday Night Fever* to enjoy the social and health benefits of dancing. Many people find dancing to be much more fun and fluid under the influence of cannabis. This is why it has been used in religious rituals for thousands of years, and why it is so popular at concerts. Cannabis helps people feel less self-conscious and more flexible, making it easier for them to lose themselves and feel more in touch with their bodies. Of course, if you take too high a dose, it might have the opposite effect and make you feel anxious and self-conscious.

## INSIGHTS AND PERCEPTIONS

One of the oddest yet most valuable effects of cannabis is that it can change the content of your thinking. Cannabis can facilitate introspection. People can gain profoundly valuable insights about themselves, their relationships, their work, their creative projects, other people, and life itself, while under the influence. I truly believe that this property of cannabis has the potential to help people learn and grow. I have seen this time and again. Not every insight is useful, of course—some can be quite fanciful and trivial—but others can be accurate and helpful. It's not likely that one would have those insights without using cannabis. Carl Sagan has discussed how cannabis helped facilitate his scientific process, writing: "I am convinced that the devastating insights achieved when high are real insights; the main problem is putting these insights in a form acceptable to the quite different self that we are when we're down the next day."[5]

My strategy has always been to write down my insights—that's how I get them into a form that is useful the next day. When the effects of cannabis have worn off, I edit them and discard the ones that are nonsense. In a fascinating passage, below, from Carl Sagan's Pulitzer Prize–winning book *The Dragons of Eden*, Sagan speculates on how, essentially, "stoned thinking" comes about.

> Our awareness of right hemisphere function is a little like our ability to see stars in the daytime. The sun is so bright that the stars are invisible, despite the fact that they are just as present as they are in the daytime as at night. When the sun sets, we are able to perceive the stars. In the same way, the brilliance of our most recent evolutionary accretion, the verbal abilities of the left hemisphere, obscures our awareness of the functions of the intuitive

> right hemisphere, which in our ancestors must have been the principal means of perceiving the world. . . . Marijuana is often described as improving our appreciation of and abilities in music, dance, art, pattern and sign recognition and our sensitivity to nonverbal communication. . . . I wonder if, rather than enhancing anything, the cannabinols . . . simply suppress the left hemisphere and permit the stars to come out.[6]

In other words, cannabis can help us to temporarily access different parts of our brain that help us with insight and other faculties. This likely occurs at the transient expense of other faculties, such as short-term memory. This is not unlike how psychedelic drugs work (see chapter 9)—by facilitating different parts of the brain to interact in novel ways.

## BOREDOM

One very common reason people use cannabis is to alleviate the boredom of the day-to-day. One could argue that all of us should be able to tolerate boredom without a drug—it is an intrinsic part of our lives, after all, and it shouldn't be necessary to medicate it. I couldn't agree more with that point of view and think it is especially relevant to teens, who need to stay away from cannabis and learn how to deal with "life on life's terms." Instead of escaping with cannabis, they need to develop "distress tolerance" and learn how to "self-soothe," skills that will help them throughout their lives.

That said, there are many older people who are facing a lot of drudgery, loneliness, and boredom in their lives. For them, there are too many hours in the day that need to be filled, now that they have fewer friends—or opportunities to participate in activities they used to enjoy—and more physical limitations. You can only spend so much time reading, chatting on the phone, or watching TV. Cannabis can make daily life more fun and tolerable.

It can even make everyday tasks more interesting. For example, folding laundry, cleaning the house, or organizing a closet is about as boring as it gets (in my opinion). When you perform these activities after using cannabis, however, they can become much more fun. You might find yourself putting on music and singing and dancing around while you're doing chores that would be dull otherwise. Cannabis can give you a feeling of youthful enthusiasm and the energy of a teenager, with nothing but adventure in front of you. This may sound silly if you've never tried it, but cannabis truly can help you get into a "flow state." It can make mundane tasks a lot more enjoyable, or at least less miserable, and you might have interesting and helpful thoughts at the same time. Even better, you can share cannabis with a friend and get through your chores together as a fun way to help each other out.

## SOCIAL CONNECTION

In our society, aging can include a lot of separation, loss, and social isolation. It has been described as an "epidemic of loneliness." It is estimated that one in three elderly people suffer from loneliness. I suspect that the real number is much higher. To fix this, we would need to make massive changes to our country's social safety net so that people don't have to worry about money and health care during their final days; and we need a thorough rethinking of how we house our elders, as well as how we deal with death and dying. With more communal living, fewer people would rot away in isolated homes they can no longer afford or be relegated to substandard nursing homes.

Though it's not a panacea, cannabis can help alleviate some of the symptoms of society's failure to meet the needs of our elderly. It can provide a shared, communal activity, and as an intellectual and social lubricant, it can make get-togethers livelier. Humans have been using cannabis for exactly that purpose for thousands of years.

Cannabis is a safer and healthier alternative to alcohol, which many people use for the sad purpose of numbing the pain of their loneliness. Alcohol has many more health harms and risks than cannabis and can act as a central nervous system depressant. It can worsen one's mood and one's sleep. As discussed in chapter 5, using cannabis is not risk free, but it is generally less harmful than using other drugs and alcohol. As added bonuses, cannabis won't give you much of a hangover, if you have one at all, the next day, and it doesn't have any carbohydrates or calories.

## A DETAILED STUDY ON LIFESTYLE BENEFITS

The war on drugs strongly discouraged any research into the beneficial effects of cannabis, as it was solely focused on tainting and demonizing it. I have been criticized for speaking about some of the nonmedical benefits of cannabis. From time to time, some ancient doctor who didn't get the memo yet that our society, by and large, now accepts the use of cannabis, accuses me of "promoting cannabis use." Once, I even got shouted down while I was giving a "grand rounds" talk at a prestigious academic medical center. I don't understand this criticism. We can't possibly understand cannabis if we don't discuss all aspects of it—the good as well as the bad. We don't create the positives of cannabis use by discussing them; their benefits have been known for thousands of years. We just allow people to make informed decisions.

One fascinating study squeaked through before Richard Nixon started his massive propaganda campaign against cannabis. This study investigated purely recreational uses of cannabis by giving cannabis users detailed surveys. The results shine light on the different ways in which cannabis can enhance one's lifestyle, consistent with what was discussed above, beyond just alleviating symptoms. These responses also can give insight into what it feels like to be "high" for people who are curious, but who have never experienced it.[7] Although the study surveyed younger people, older Americans also experienced the results:

> Visual effects were sharpened—"I can see new colors or more subtle shades of color."
>
> Auditory effects were deepened—"The notes of music are purer and more distinct. "
>
> Touch effects were heightened—"My sense of touch is more exciting, more sensual. "
>
> Taste effects were enhanced—"Taste sensations take on new qualities. . . . I crave sweet things to eat, like chocolate."
>
> Space-time perception was changed—"Time passes very slowly."
>
> Body perception was changed—"I feel a lot of pleasant warmth inside my body."
>
> Interpersonal experiences were changed—"I empathize tremendously with others; I feel what they feel . . ."
>
> Sexual experiences were affected—"Sexual orgasm has new qualities, pleasurable qualities; when making love, I feel like I'm in much closer mental contact with my partner; it's much more of a union of souls as well as bodies."
>
> Thought processes were changed —"I give little or no thought to the future; I am completely in the here-and-

> now," " The ideas that come to my mind are much more original," . . . "I have more imagery than usual when I'm reading—images of the scene I'm reading about just pop up vividly."[8]

This study is thought-provoking, as it is one of the few to assess the experience of cannabis use without an a priori agenda of making it sound scary or harmful.

In theory, a drug- and medicine-free world might be healthier, but that is not the world we live in. Virtually all societies throughout history have used intoxicants. In a perfect world, we'd exercise, meditate, eat tofu, go to therapy, do yoga, participate in classes, etc., to stay relaxed, happy, and pain free. In that scenario, we would be healthy and content, and few of us would need anything to "take the edge off," even as we age and accumulate diagnoses.

In the world we actually live in, however, many if not most people need something, in addition to their medical regimen, at the end of the day. Traditionally, the one legal option has been alcohol. For decades, we have been bombarded with advertisements to make us think that we like and need it. We have been conditioned to crave alcohol regardless of whether we actually enjoy its effects. Advertising works. In reality, alcohol is increasingly viewed as carcinogenic. In 2024, it was a factor in an estimated 178,000 alcohol-related deaths.[9] As cannabis is becoming legal, state by state, it is no wonder that people, young and old alike, are pivoting toward cannabis.

With some modest education, people can learn to use cannabis safely and effectively, whether it is strictly for medical uses or for lifestyle enhancement.

CHAPTER 9

# How Psychedelic Drugs Might Help

Psychedelic drugs change one's mood, perceptions, and sensations. They are also called hallucinogens. They change how we think, and they can help different parts of our brains communicate with each other in new ways. These drugs/medicines can get us out of negative, unhelpful thought patterns, such as ruminations, and have been used recreationally for decades and in religious ceremonies for millennia. Like cannabis, they are enjoying a resurgence of interest among patients, researchers, and doctors alike. These days, when you tune into the news it is hard not to hear about psilocybin (magic mushrooms or shrooms), LSD (acid), MDMA (Ecstasy), ketamine, and other psychedelic drugs. The most popular stories tend to highlight extreme cases—both miraculous cures and scary "bad trips"—because clickbait attracts attention. But there is a lot more to know about these emerging medicines that goes beyond sensational stories.

## HOW CAN PSYCHEDELICS HELP, AND WHAT ARE THE RISKS?

Even though cannabis can have psychedelic properties when taken in high doses, psychedelics are in a separate class. The psychoactive effects of psychedelic drugs, at standard doses, are far stronger than cannabis, and can initiate a "trip" that profoundly affects your perception of reality for many hours at a time. For psychiatric purposes, these drugs are most beneficial when used with the help of a psychedelic guide or therapist who can make the experience more long lastingly therapeutic—and safe. Psychedelics work in a couple of ways: They make a patient's brain and personality more open to therapy and helpful suggestions for a brief time after their use, and they promote neuroplasticity by helping the brain form new types of connections.

The "trip" one experiences on psychedelics can be profoundly pleasurable and meaningful or terrifying and upsetting, depending on a number of factors, including the "set and setting" (see pages 229–231). Set and setting are critical, as it is important that you use psychedelics in an appropriate and relaxing setting, away from adult responsibilities. Unless you are extremely experienced with psychedelics, it is best to take a trip with a "trip sitter," someone who accompanies you but does not take the drug. As of this writing, psychedelics are not yet legal yet in the United States, except in a few states (Oregon, Colorado, and, recently, New Mexico). If you would like to try psychedelics, which many people are eager to do, you must either sign up for a study at an academic medical center or go to a state—or another country—where psychedelics are legal. Alternatively, you can go underground and use the "gray" market to find a practitioner. The services they provide, however, can be unregulated and not entirely legal or safe.

Most people tend to use psychedelics intermittently because trips are so intense, and it takes a while to assimilate and recover from them. However, some people use psychedelic drugs daily, by "microdosing" them, which means taking a tiny dose—not enough to feel the effects, but enough, potentially, to harness some of the drug's benefits. For example, they might take a dose of psilocybin (the active ingredient in psilocybin-containing mushrooms) every day, in a quantity so small that they wouldn't have any perceptual distortions, to reduce anxiety and increase creativity. Many people swear by microdosing, although there isn't much scientific evidence to support this practice. Some drugs, such as ketamine, are often taken periodically, often through injections, to sustain their therapeutic benefit.

Psychedelic drugs are being investigated as potentially game-changing treatments for conditions such as chronic pain, treatment-resistant depression, OCD (obsessive-compulsive disorder), trauma, cluster headaches, and substance misuse. Psychedelics are also proving to be highly effective in alleviating the fear of death, anxiety, and suffering experienced by people who are receiving end-of-life care or who have a terminal medical condition.

This chapter will explore the exciting new research in the field of "classic" psychedelic drugs such as psilocybin and LSD, as well as "atypical" psychedelics, such as MDMA and ketamine.

## WHY DO PEOPLE USE PSYCHEDELIC DRUGS?

Many people use psychedelics to enhance their enjoyment of other people and nature, and to delve more deeply into their spirituality. Others use psychedelics to better understand themselves and their wants and needs—or to boost creativity. If used safely, psychedelics can be an interesting and helpful counterbalance to the daily drudgery of normal life and can result in lasting improvements in how you view the world and relate to other people.

Medically, the most common reasons people use psychedelics are to tackle treatment-resistant depression; work through trauma and PTSD; address end-of-life concerns, such as fear of death; and help treat conditions like OCD and addiction.

## Treatment-Resistant Depression

When a patient is severely depressed and hasn't had a significant response to conventional treatments, such as antidepressants, they are considered to be "treatment resistant." Under those circumstances, people suffer immensely and can become hopeless and suicidal. Researchers have found that several psychedelic drugs, such as psilocybin and ketamine,[1] can break through seemingly unsurmountable depression and provide rapid relief. Although further study and confirmation are needed, the initial results are inspiring a lot of hope.

## Addiction

The use of psychedelics is showing great potential for treating addiction, including addiction to alcohol.[2] Bill Wilson, the founder of the recovery group AA (Alcoholics Anonymous), was public about how he used LSD to achieve the spiritual awakening that allowed him to enter into remission from alcohol use disorder.[3] (One may reasonably question why the group he formed is so rigidly focused on absolute abstinence when its founder used a drug to get into recovery!) Ketamine and psilocybin have shown positive results. Ibogaine, a psychedelic herb that comes from the bark of a Central African shrub, is purported to be extremely effective in helping people get over opioid addiction, although it might not be as safe as other psychedelic drugs given its potentially dangerous effects on the heart.

## OCD (Obsessive-Compulsive Disorder)

Obsessive-compulsive disorder is a mental health condition in which the patient suffers frequent unwanted thoughts, ruminations, and obsessions that cause compulsive behavior, including repetitive behavior that can negatively affect social interactions and everyday activities. Mainstream medications for this condition, primarily Prozac, offer some, but not complete, relief. Many anecdotal reports of different psychedelic drugs that can help people with symptoms of OCD are being researched.[4]

## Trauma and PTSD (Post-Traumatic Stress Disorder)

The health and psychological effects of trauma are devastating. Many cases of addiction and depression are influenced by adverse childhood experiences or other traumas, such as those suffered by military veterans. All psychedelics have some potential to help with trauma and with the symptoms of PTSD. One psychedelic, MDMA, commonly known as ecstasy or molly, has garnered most of the attention; it is best used along with therapy. According to one study, "These data suggest that MDMA-AT [MDMA-Assisted Therapy] reduced PTSD symptoms and functional impairment in a diverse population with moderate to severe PTSD and was generally well tolerated."[5] MDMA can help people process traumatic memories and events in a way that makes them less painful, threatening, and disruptive.

Ibogaine has recently garnered a tremendous amount of attention, especially among combat veterans who are trying to treat their trauma histories. As of this writing, the state of Texas just approved $50 million for research into how ibogaine treatment can help combat veterans recover from their trauma.

## End-of-Life Care

A recent *New York Times* article discussed in detail how psychedelics—specifically, psilocybin and ketamine—are helping people accept and adjust to the idea of dying as they approach the end of their life.[6] Psychedelics can help alleviate the pain, anxiety, and dread that usually come along with this stage of life. Although psychedelics have rarely been studied specifically in older patients, one study found that using classic psychedelics like psilocybin and LSD helped reduce anxiety and depression in patients with life-threatening diseases (e.g., cancer). The study also found that "existential distress (such as feeling that life has no meaning) and quality of life may be improved" with the use of classic psychedelics. The authors of the study emphasize that although the data base they used is small and incomplete, it has intriguing potential for future research and clinical application.[7]

Another study also reported that "psychedelics, especially psilocybin and LSD, showed promising effects on depression and anxiety in people with terminal illnesses."[8] In comparison, the traditional medications we use for these conditions, such as opioids and benzodiazepines, are only somewhat effective—they are comparable to clubbing a patient senseless—and have serious side effects, such as sedation, nausea and vomiting, and constipation, not to mention the risks associated with long-term use.

Due to the results of studies like the ones I just cited, and others like them, there has been a tremendous resurgence of interest in the potential use of psychedelics in palliative care. The initial results suggest that psychedelics can provide lasting benefits. A recent study of people with cancer and depression found that 80 percent of patients who took a single dose of psilocybin had a sustained, positive response, and that 50 percent reported full remission in depressive symptoms two months later.[9]

Finally, another study, cited below, not only observed that "psilocybin-assisted psychotherapy holds promise in promoting long-term relief from cancer-related psychiatric distress," but also showed that the benefits were durable.

> At the second (4.5 year) follow-up approximately 60–80 percent of participants met criteria for clinically significant antidepressant or anxiolytic responses. Participants overwhelmingly (71–100 percent) attributed positive life changes to the psilocybin-assisted therapy experience and rated it among the most personally meaningful and spiritually significant experiences of their lives.[10]

End-of-life and palliative care, hospice, cancer, fear of death, trauma, depression—the use of psychedelics in all of these areas needs to be researched further. Initial indications are that psychedelics have the profound potential to help alleviate some of the worst fears and discomforts that inevitably arise for all of us as we get closer to the end of life.

## HOW DO PSYCHEDELICS WORK?

Although researchers are still trying to understand how psychedelics can help alleviate existential distress, depression, pain, and addiction, we know exactly which serotonin receptors in the brain are affected by them. SSRIs—drugs such as fluoxetine (Prozac), paroxetine (Paxil), sertraline (Zoloft), citalopram (Celexa)—work to alleviate depression and anxiety in an analogous way, because they interact with some of the same serotonin receptors.

Without knowing exactly how psychedelics work, we have seen how helpful they can be in reducing circular, pessimistic, and ruminative thinking, which is often a critical component of mental illness. We worry about things we have no control over, and we ruminate endlessly, much to our detriment. This "stinking thinking" harms our moods. Unhelpful neuronal pathways become worn into our brain, like goat paths, by these unhelpful modes of thinking. However, we believe that psychedelics can help in a variety of ways, including by doing these four things:

1. **Reboot Your Brain:** When you take a psychedelic, there is less blood flow to the DFN (default mode network), the part of the brain that is engaged during quiet wakefulness, and that allows us to experience feelings associated with daydreaming and self-reflection. Instead, blood flow is redirected to different parts of the brain, allowing them to communicate with each other more then they ordinarily do. This activity helps to ameliorate negative, ruminative thoughts by supplanting them with newer, healthier ways to view the world.
2. **Promote Neuroplasticity:** Neuroplasticity is the brain's ability to reorganize its functions, connections, and structures, in response to new experiences and stimuli. Psychedelics promote neuroplasticity and therefore are helpful in forming new ways to think and feel about the world and relationships. This rewiring of the brain, induced by psychedelics, allows patients to see their lives and struggles from a fresh vantage point and helps to heal the brain from past traumas.
3. **Assist Psychiatric Therapy:** It isn't just psychedelic drugs themselves that are thought to be so helpful in treating psychiatric conditions; rather, it is psychedelic-assisted therapy that provides the greatest benefit. In psychedelic-assisted therapy, patients are prepped for the experience beforehand by a guide or therapist. Soon after their trip, they typically "integrate" the experience in intensive therapy sessions. Patients are particularly amenable and open to therapy in the weeks that follow a psychedelic experience and tend to make great progress.

4. **Experience the Mystical:** When people take a regular to large dose of a psychedelic, they often hallucinate and experience deeply spiritual and, at times, out-of-body experiences. This mystical occurrence is thought to contribute to the growth and change that can come with taking psychedelics. Some drug companies are investigating the possibility of developing psychedelics that can deliver the same benefits of taking the drug without the trip. My suspicion is that the mystical aspect of the experience will prove to be the crucial component for making psychological progress.

## HOW TO CONSUME PSYCHEDELICS

There are two ways to consume psychedelics: regular dosing, where you take enough of the drug to alter thoughts and perceptions; and microdosing, where you can get the benefits of psychedelics, such as improved mood, energy, and creativity, without hallucinating or being spaced out and incapacitated for many hours. People can go to work and drive after microdosing—they won't be impaired (unless they've miscalculated the dose).

Microdosing is currently exceedingly popular with hundreds of thousands of people who tout its benefits. The evidence base is mixed, however, and it has not yet been definitively determined by scientific studies whether microdosing truly works as advertised, or if it works by placebo effect. In any case, microdosing involves taking a minuscule dosage of a psychedelic drug—typically one-twentieth to one-fifth of a regular dose. With that small a dose, you won't experience hallucinations or perceptual distortions, assuming you haven't made a mistake with the dose. The multitude of people who are microdosing are absolutely convinced that by taking small doses of psychedelics they are improving mood, energy, and creativity. I wouldn't be surprised if science catches up to their claims and confirms the benefits.

## CLASSIC PSYCHEDELICS

All psychedelic drugs categorized as classic interact with the same serotonin receptor in the brain, which is why they all have somewhat similar effects. But each drug has unique qualities and provides distinct experiences, due to differences in exactly *how* it interacts with the serotonin receptor. The classic psychedelics are profiled here and below through page 225.

### Psilocybin

Also known as magic mushrooms or shrooms, fungi containing psilocybin widely used recreationally as well as medically. Using them recreationally, I've found them to be fun, mind-expanding, and meaningful. For example, after eating shrooms and taking a walk in the woods with friends, I found that both my relationship with my friends and the way I view colors in the natural world were permanently affected for the better. The only bad part of the experience is the disgusting taste of the mushrooms, although some fans might not be bothered by it. An initial episode of nausea can be a side effect of magic mushrooms. The dosage is very variable—it depends on how strong the shrooms are, and what type of effect you are looking for (e.g., taking just a little can impart a magical feeling, while taking a larger dose can lead to a full-blown mystical experience; therapeutic doses tend to be in between the two). A mushroom trip might last for around four hours, although one's sense of time is somewhat distorted. In any case, you'll remember the entire trip.

Shrooms are being studied to treat difficult-to-manage conditions, such as treatment-resistant depression, alcoholism, cluster headaches, and OCD, with promising initial results. They also appear to be particularly helpful for end-of-life care.

### LSD (Lysergic Acid Diethylamide)

The term "LSD" is an acronym for the chemical name of the drug lysergic acid diethylamide. It is commonly referred to by its street name, "acid," and is a liquid that is often added to absorbent or "blotter" paper cut into small squares, or sold in micro-tablets. This drug, along with cannabis, is a big part of what fueled the cultural explosion of the 1960s. It can cause profound perceptual distortions and can be quite scary if taken in too high a dosage or if taken in the wrong setting. It lasts for a long time—about eight hours. Unless you've had a lot of experience with psychedelics, it's best to take LSD in a controlled, therapeutic setting.

The main medical uses of LSD are for anxiety, depression, and addiction. In 2024, the FDA (Federal Drug Administration) granted breakthrough therapy designation to LSD for the treatment of generalized anxiety disorder. According to one article, "This decision follows a landmark study indicating that a single dose of the drug could offer lasting relief to individuals grappling with this debilitating condition."[11] Despite the FDA's historic acknowledgment of the therapeutic aspect of LSD, however, it is still inexplicably relegated to Schedule I of the Controlled Substance Act, which specifies that LSD has no medical benefit and high misuse liability (neither is accurate). Recent studies of LSD suggest promising results.

### DMT (Dimethyltryptamine)/Ayahuasca

DMT is the active ingredient in ayahuasca, an herbal brew that has been used for centuries in South America for healing and divination. It is a profoundly intense and immersive trip that can last for up to twelve hours. This powerful hallucinogen should be used only by extremely experienced users of psychedelics, under careful supervision. People who go through ayahuasca experiences often claim that it helps them with depression, anxiety, and addiction, and, most particularly, with overcoming past traumatic experiences.

If you choose to take a psychedelic that is as strong and mind-bending as DMT, you absolutely need a guide to help you. For that reason, many people go on "ayahuasca retreats," but be aware that they are unregulated and should be thoroughly researched and vetted to make sure they are safe. It is critical to be an informed consumer in these situations if you want to find a place that is reputable. There are competent, safe places, but you have to do some legwork to find them.

## Peyote/Mescaline

Mescaline is a psychedelic drug that occurs naturally in the peyote cactus as well as in several other cacti species. Peyote, which is native to northern Mexico and southwestern Texas, has been used by Indigenous peoples in America for sacramental ceremonies and healing for centuries. It is an integral part of religious practice in the NAC (Native American Church), which was founded in the late nineteenth century. The peyote supply is severely limited, however, because of habitat loss and unsustainable and negligent harvesting—not only by those in the illegal drug trade, but by "psychedelic tourists" (novelty-seeking drugs users) as well. The NAC respectfully requests that the currently available peyote supply be reserved for the traditional uses of their members.[12] Everyone needs to respect this request.

## ATYPICAL PSYCHEDELICS

Atypical psychedelics are a diverse set of drugs and medicines. They work on a variety of different receptor systems through mechanisms that are different from the serotonin receptors used by classic psychedelics. They can have a wide range of effects and uses. There is incredible excitement about the therapeutic potential of these drugs.

### Ketamine

Ketamine was approved for clinical use in the US in 1970 and is still used as a surgical and veterinary anesthetic. Powdered Ketamine emerged as a recreational drug at around the same time and became known as "Vitamin K" in the 1980s. Ketamine then became further popularized as a party drug in the 1990s under the moniker "Special K," due to its ability to cause euphoria and dissociation. It has now become increasingly sought after for a variety of mental health conditions, such as TRD (treatment-resistant depression), alcoholism, and anxiety. Ketamine is also used in many hospitals and ketamine clinics and can be sourced legally via mail-order suppliers.

Ketamine clinics, which are sprouting up all over the place, typically provide an injection or an infusion of the drug. They might also provide esketamine (Spravato), a ketamine nasal spray that was approved by the FDA for use in treating depression in 2019. After receiving a dose of ketamine in a clinic—whether it is an intravenous injection, constitutes a shot in the arm, or is taken intranasally—you must be observed and supported for several hours. This is done to make sure you don't have any adverse effects to the drug or do anything dangerous as a result of the profound dissociation it brings on. Ketamine treatment requires a substantial time commitment. It is also expensive and, unfortunately, spottily covered by insurance.

Many hospitals now have ketamine clinics where they monitor and treat people, but waiting lists for this popular therapy tend to be long. Mail-order suppliers of ketamine can also send you small ketamine-impregnated wafers or "troches." These lozenges dissolve slowly in your mouth and provide a lower dosage than one you might get at a ketamine clinic. People find lozenges exceedingly effective. Recently, one supplier started sending injectable ketamine kits through the mail. Ketamine is particularly effective for the alleviation of treatment-resistant depression. TRD is a cruel condition that is diagnosed when a person with severe depression has not shown improvement after taking various traditional antidepressants, such as SSRIs, or undergoing other treatments, such as electroconvulsive therapy. The risk of suicide can be quite high among patients who suffer from TRD. After receiving ketamine, however, some people have reported that their depression lifts in about forty minutes. Often, these are the same people who have been battling depression for years or decades. Although this may sound too good to be true, it is well supported by data. Ketamine is also being investigated for its potential to help relieve pain and symptoms of OCD. Ketamine is generally considered to be safe if medically monitored, even for those who are experiencing suicidal thoughts.

The main side effects of ketamine can be intoxication, sedation, euphoria, high blood pressure, dizziness, headache, blurred vision, bladder irritation, anxiety, and nausea. At higher doses, ketamine can cause a profound disconnection from reality. This is called "disassociation," which is a weird and potentially dangerous thing to experience if it is not monitored in a safe setting. An overdose of ketamine can cause unconsciousness and dangerously slowed breathing, and can be fatal, especially if mixed with alcohol.

Ketamine needs to be taken under safe circumstances, with a good deal of monitoring, preparation, and knowledge of its effects. As with all other psychedelics, Ketamine is most effective when it is given in the context of "assisted therapy," rather than just taking the drug on your own. Ketamine hasn't been studied specifically for use in the elderly, but I think it is safe to say that it should be used with particular caution if there is a history of dementia, confusion, falls, or liver or kidney disease.

## MDMA (Ecstasy)

Methylenedioxymethamphetamine or MDMA has been a popular party drug for decades due to its ability to produce euphoria; increase energy; and facilitate empathy, sexuality, and compassion. In the 1970s, MDMA was investigated, with extremely promising results, by psychiatrists, who believed it could help treat trauma and also help married couples navigate their difficulties with connection while in therapy. Then, due to the federal government's war on drugs, almost all research on MDMA was stopped in the 1980s, over the outcry of psychiatrists. Now, interest in this drug has reemerged, and research is firing on all cylinders.

MDMA is currently being studied to help alleviate PTSD and trauma, as well as other conditions, such as alcoholism. In 2017, the FDA granted breakthrough therapy designation to MDMA-assisted psychotherapy for the treatment of PTSD, which was particularly momentous because of the paucity of effective medical treatments for this condition.

With MDMA, people can experience side effects including low sodium (hyponatremia) and dehydration, as well as an elevated body temperature (hyperthermia). They can also develop "serotonin syndrome"—too much serotonin, which causes flushing, diarrhea, and high blood pressure—if they take it with the wrong drug (such as an SSRI). Other side effects include blurred vision, bruxism (teeth grinding), insomnia, rapid heart rate, and a rebound of sadness and lethargy in the days after MDMA use, referred to as "Blue Monday."

Use of atypical psychedelics such as MDMA and ketamine can also lead to addiction, although not nearly at the levels seen with alcohol or opioids. Any drug that causes euphoria can trigger addiction in people who are susceptible. This is especially true of MDMA, which is why it is called "ecstasy." Only a small percentage of people get addicted to ketamine. Classic psychedelics, such as shrooms/psilocybin or LSD, are not considered to be addictive.

One last nonclassic drug to mention is ibogaine, which comes from the *Tabernanthe iboga* shrub, native to Central Africa. Ibogaine has been called the Mount Everest of psychedelic drugs, and its all-encompassing effects can last for twenty-four hours. There is tremendous interest in using ibogaine to treat addiction and trauma. However, one must be mindful of the drug's side effects, including potentially fatal heart arrhythmias, and difficulty coping with the length and intensity of the trip itself.

## WHAT CAN GO WRONG WHEN USING PSYCHEDELIC DRUGS?

No drug or medication, however "natural" or popular, is without risks and adverse effects. This is a significant concern with classic psychedelics, which can so profoundly alter one's consciousness. Although most people tend to have pleasurable, interesting, and helpful experiences with psychedelics that border on the mystical, a certain percentage, perhaps 10 percent, have "bad trips." These can be terrifying and lead to a panic attack or even send you to the ER. Some people have lasting trauma from these experiences. Interestingly, one study revealed that 84 percent of people who have had bad trips still view the experience as a positive one that results in growth and change.[13] That said, bad trips are still to be avoided to the greatest possible extent. After all, there are ways to set yourself up for success.

The risk of having a bad trip is greatly minimized if you arrange to have the experience in a restful and safe "set and setting," without the intrusion of complex or challenging social interactions. It is of utmost importance to be in a relaxing, peaceful environment—out in nature, for example, or even at home, listening to some quiet music—where you can consume the drug without being called upon to deal with a stressful work or childcare emergency. That's why it is so important to plan a trip beforehand. Remember, too, that you must not operate machinery or drive under the influence of a psychedelic drug.

It is imperative to take a reasonable dosage of psychedelics—nothing "heroic," especially when you are just starting out. Very high doses of psychedelics can result in a scary, strange experience that causes anxiety and depersonalization. Because there is always the risk of having an unpleasant or uncomfortable experience, it is recommended that you have someone with you who is sober, and who can soothe and calm you. On the rare occasion when that type of reassurance doesn't work and things continue to escalate, you might need to visit the ER. A longer-term side effect of psychedelics can include lasting perceptual distortions, known as HPPD (hallucinogen persisting perceptual disorder). In this situation, people experience disturbing flashbacks for years. Although that side effect is rare, it is uncomfortable and destabilizing.

Certain drugs and medicines can interact with psychedelics to blunt their effects. If you are taking an SSRI, classic psychedelics might not do much—there'll be no trip, few perceptual changes, and little psychological benefit. That's because the drugs are competing for the same serotonin receptors in your brain. There is also the possibility of getting too much serotonin activation or serotonin syndrome (see page 228), causing confusion and agitation. The atypical psychedelic MDMA also has little to no effect if a person is on an SSRI, whereas ketamine is not impacted by the use of SSRIs or other antidepressants.

Legality is an issue with psychedelic drugs, even though several of them have been granted breakthrough therapy designation by the FDA in order to facilitate research. Other than ketamine, all psychedelic drugs are federally illegal in the United States, except in certain research settings. As of this writing, three states have legalized psychedelics: Colorado, Oregon, and New Mexico. As with all illegal drugs, the illegality of psychedelics makes them that much more dangerous. It can be difficult to obtain a safe supply of a drug that is illegal. It is even harder to ask for help, due to fear and stigma. The illegality of drugs drives them underground and makes it difficult for patients to discuss the possibility of using them with their doctors. Fortunately, there is bipartisan political momentum for lessening the restrictions on the use of psychedelics, both on a federal level and in many states. As mentioned previously, beware of psychedelic "retreats," as many of them are unregulated, are of substandard quality, and could be downright dangerous.

Psychedelic drugs should always be used under medical supervision, or in a very carefully thought-out setting—if they're used at all. The right dose, a competent "trip sitter," a safe supply, and the proper mindset and environment—set and setting—are the keys to a successful experience. It is a good idea to speak with your physician about using psychedelics to make sure it is safe, given any medical conditions you may have.

# Afterword

As a primary care physician for a quarter century, and as a longstanding cannabis specialist, I have seen many harms wrought by excessive or inappropriate cannabis use. I have seen severe cases of cannabis addiction and have dealt with people who have psychosis that was either caused or worsened by cannabis. I have had patients with hyperemesis (extreme vomiting from cannabis use) and patients who puff on vapes uncontrollably, every fifteen minutes, to the detriment of their lungs—and to the point where it is unlikely that there are any benefits from use. I also know of people who have passed out after taking a hit from a joint. Cannabis is not harm-free and must be used cautiously and mindfully, as is the case with any drug or medicine.

Most of us have learned about cannabis in the context of the war on drugs, which was launched in 1971 and is still ongoing, more than fifty years later. The use of cannabis was deliberately tainted and stigmatized, particularly in the early years of the "war," via a massive propaganda campaign that painted cannabis as far more harmful than it really is. All of that has made it exceedingly difficult to have a sensible discussion about the actual harms and medical benefits of cannabis. Doctors and patients are divided into camps that are unreasonably for or against cannabis, when the truth is often found somewhere in the middle.

It is critical for all of us to learn how to speak about both the positives and negatives of cannabis use. On the one hand, prohibitionists tend to minimize and gloss over the obvious medicinal and lifestyle benefits of cannabis; on the other hand, cannabis enthusiasts often downplay many of the potential harms of cannabis use, such as addiction and deleterious effects on pregnancy. Surely, by this point in time, we should be able to agree on some common ground. We should all be able to agree that cannabis helps with pain, anxiety, and insomnia, and with the side effects of chemotherapy, and that it is dangerous in pregnancy, psychosis, cardiac patients, and for teens.

I have always been opposed to criminalizing behaviors that people are going to do anyway, which clearly has been the case with cannabis. Doing so makes the entire enterprise more hazardous. It results in a more dangerous product and needless arrests, predominantly of Black and Hispanic people, due to the well-documented racist enforcement of cannabis laws. There have been twenty million arrests for nonviolent cannabis use over the last half century to no purpose, which has caused great hardship.[1] Criminalization also denies people access to a medical plant that, as we have discussed, has the potential to alleviate a tremendous amount of suffering. Few would argue against the notion that our world needs less suffering.

Regarding cannabis policy, things in the United States have been heading in the right direction. Use of cannabis is now fully legal in twenty-five states in which more than half of Americans live. It is legal for medical use in thirty-nine states, with other states having provisions for CBD and very low THC. Eventually, I believe that cannabis—at least medical cannabis—will be fully legal in this country, as well as in many other countries.

On a more personal note, I have prescribed cannabis to help thousands of patients. Many are elderly and are doing better on cannabis than they were with traditional pharmaceuticals. They are experiencing fewer toxicities and side effects. Cannabis prescription is helping with polypharmacy. Patients are getting vitally needed relief in a way that wasn't available to them without medical cannabis. Their health-related quality of life is improving. Cannabis certainly isn't for everyone. For some patients it does not work, and in others, it can have noxious side effects. Some people greatly dislike the psychoactive effect of cannabis. The results are highly personalized, as is the best dose. We can never know if it might be helpful until a patient tries it.

I started treating patients several decades before most doctors believed in medical marijuana. I am profoundly grateful that the medical profession is finally embracing cannabis as a helpful medicine. When I started out, most of my colleagues were skeptical. In the year 2000, when I was a medical resident, I gave my senior presentation on medical cannabis at Harvard's Brigham and Women's Hospital. The other residents were vaguely supportive, and, being of a younger generation, they weren't particularly opposed to it. Still, they were quite skeptical and somewhat indifferent. Now, some of those same physicians are referring patients to me.

Most doctors are now in favor of medical cannabis. One challenge is that, even if they are supporters, they haven't been taught much practical knowledge with which to guide patients. Younger doctors, particularly interns and residents, are particularly bitter about this. We owe it to our patients, as a profession, to get up to speed quickly on this issue, and in such a fashion that we can meet them halfway.

It is difficult to overstate the effect that my late father, the legendary Harvard psychiatrist Dr. Lester Grinspoon, had on all of this. His 1971 masterpiece, *Marihuana Reconsidered*, provided ample intellectual firepower for the cannabis legalization movement. It helped counter the lies and misrepresentations coming from the US government as it peddled its poisonous and dishonest war on drugs. My father's 1993 book, *Marihuana: The Forbidden Medicine*, educated and inspired thousands of doctors and patients alike. It paved the way for California to become the first state to legalize medical marijuana in 1996. I remember seeing a photograph of my father on the front page of the *Boston Globe* in 2018, forty-seven years after *Marihuana Reconsidered* came out, smoking the first legally sold joint in his home state of Massachusetts. After a half-century of advocacy, he was winning the war.

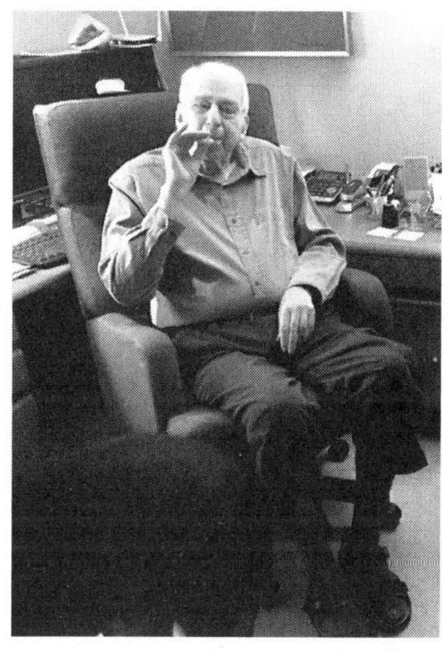

**Dr. Lester Grinspoon, shown here in a detail of a photograph from the *Boston Globe* cover story of December 21, 2018, entitled: "What Happened to the First Recreational Pot Sold in Mass?"**

Like my patients, I have had helpful experiences with medical cannabis. I first experimented with cannabis at age thirteen—which I don't recommend. Like many teens, my thirteen-year-old self was more interested in novelty-seeking than in common sense. As an adult, I find cannabis helps with pain, anxiety, and sleep. It was particularly useful in treating the blistering migraines I would get as an intern and a resident after a thirty-six-hour shift in the hospital. Nothing else worked. Yet, with one puff, the migraine drifted away. I was able to enjoy the evening, recharge my batteries, sleep, and function the next day.

Cannabis also helped me transition away from taking prescription opioids during my destructive opioid addiction twenty years ago. It was the only thing that could alleviate the miserable withdrawal symptoms, which included aches, nausea, sweats, depression, anxiety, diarrhea, and stomach cramps (i.e., many of the symptoms that cannabis can help alleviate). After my spinal surgery, and after three recent surgeries for a shattered leg, cannabis helped me transition from postoperative pharmaceuticals, including opioids, much more quickly than otherwise would have been the case. Finally, and most impactfully, cannabis has given me so many personal insights over the decades that I truly feel it has helped make me a more compassionate, sensitive, and grounded person.

Medical cannabis is an ancient but powerful tool that is increasingly available in our modern world to alleviate suffering. We can use it to help treat some of the most excruciating problems that come with growing older and to help people with the very miseries that come with aging, such as chronic pain, anxiety, insomnia, boredom, and insomnia. We can help dying patients. We can help patients suffering from cancer or MS. The improvement in quality of life can be transformative for those who benefit from medical cannabis. This formerly forbidden medicine is rapidly coming out of the shadows and into the treatment plans of doctors and patients. Hopefully, we have given you the tools to maximize benefits, avoid harms, and improve your quality of life.

# Acknowledgments

I would like to acknowledge my innovative agent Linda Konner for giving me the idea to write this book and for helping to steer me through the complex waters of the publishing world. Thank you to my editors, Barbara Berger and Jennifer Williams, for the patient, outstanding edits and suggestions they made. Thanks also to the wonderful staff at Union Square & Co., particularly cover designer Kaylie Pendleton, interior designer Rich Hazelton, project editor Kristin Mandaglio, and production manager Sandy Noman. Thank you to my family, including my twin brother, Joshua, even though he didn't really do anything helpful, and to my brother David, who was always available for comments, ideas, encouragement, and inspiration. Thank you to Allen St. Pierre and Dr. Staci Gruber, without whom, respectively, cannabis would neither be legal nor well understood. And thank you to Dr. Gruber for her incredibly generous, heartfelt, and thoughtful foreword. Thank you to my children, Emma, Zach, and Jacob, who are so sick of hearing about this topic, generation after generation. Thank you to Jacob for helping me screw up the footnotes, using a psychotic AI system that ran amok—I couldn't have done it without you! Thank you to Benji Grinspoon and to Dr. Anthony Portnoy. Thank you to my late father, the legendary psychiatrist Dr. Lester Grinspoon, who was the intellectual backbone and leader of the cannabis legalization movement. Thank you to my mom. Not to brag, but I have the nicest mom on earth. Finally, I have sincere gratitude for my brilliant wife, Lizzi, for her kind help when I managed to destroy my computer time and time again, and for her loving encouragement and patience.

# Glossary

**Cannabinoid:** A chemical compound found in the cannabis plant that interreacts with our ECS (endocannabinoid system)

**CBD (cannabidiol):** The most abundant nonintoxicating cannabinoid found in the cannabis plant; helpful for pain, sleep, and insomnia

**CBDA:** The acidic version of CBD, used as a very strong anti-inflammatory; thought to be helpful for muscle and nerve pain

**CBN (cannabinol):** A minor cannabinoid used for sleep, as well as for pain and anxiety

**CBG (cannabigerol):** A minor cannabinoid used for muscle pain, anxiety, colitis, and to stimulate appetite

**CBC (cannabichromene):** A minor cannabinoid helpful for pain and as an anti-inflammatory

**CB1 receptor:** The first cannabinoid receptor to be discovered, found mostly in the brain and the nervous system

**CB2 receptor:** The second cannabinoid receptor, found mostly in the cells of the immune system

**Chemovar:** A more accurate word than "strain," which denotes the chemical composition of a particular type of cannabis

**CHS (cannabis hyperemesis syndrome):** A paradoxical reaction to cannabis that causes nausea, vomiting, and abdominal pain; can be experienced by heavy users

**Delta-8 THC:** A hemp-derived THC product popularly described as the mellow version of cannabis or "THC light"

**Delta-9 THC:** The chief active ingredient in cannabis; see THC

**Delta-10 THC:** A hemp-derived version of THC that is chemically similar to Delta-9 THC, which is found in cannabis

**Dry herb vaporizer:** A small device that heats up cannabis flower, which is then consumed as a vapor—and thought to be safer than smoking cannabis

**ECS (endocannabinoid system):** A system of receptors and neurotransmitters through which cannabis works its effects on our bodies

**Epidiolex:** FDA-approved prescription version of CBD

**Hemp-derived products:** Newly legalized molecules that are derived from the CBD found in hemp

**HHC:** A newly developed, highly psychoactive synthetic cannabinoid that hasn't been studied

**Indica:** A type of cannabis that is thought to be relaxing and sedating

**Minor cannabinoids:** Molecules present in the cannabis plant in smaller quantities that interact with our endocannabinoid system

**NSAIDs:** Nonsteroidal anti-inflammatory medications such as ibuprofen (Advil, Motrin), naproxen (Aleve), or diclofenac (Voltaren)

**Polypharmacy:** The simultaneous use of five or more medications

**Sativa:** A type of cannabis that is thought to be uplifting and energetic

**Strain:** A specific type of cannabis flower; strains are said to have different medicinal effects

**Synthetic cannabinoids:** Lab-made molecules that are chemically similar to the natural cannabinoids in the cannabis plants; often much stronger and more dangerous

**Terpenes:** Aromatic organic compounds found in cannabis that contribute to its smell and taste

**THC:** Delta-9 THC, the most abundant, intoxicating cannabinoid found in the cannabis plant, responsible for many of the medical benefits

**THC-O:** A new synthetic cannabinoid that is several times stronger than regular THC

**THCV (tetrahydrocannabivarin):** A minor cannabinoid that helps control appetite and blood sugar

**THC-0:** A new synthetic cannabinoid, derived from hemp

**Tincture:** A liquid version of dissolved cannabis that can be taken under the tongue

**Vape pen:** A small device that burns cannabis oil for the purpose of smoking it

# Notes


### Chapter 1: Cannabis and the Twenty-First Century: Changing Views

1 O'Shaughnessy, W. B. "On the Preparations of the Indian Hemp, or Gunjah," *Provincial Medical Journal and Retrospect of the Medical Sciences* 5 (Feb. 4, 1843): 363–369, 364, pmc.ncbi.nlm.nih.gov/articles/PMC2490264.

2 Londoño, Ernesto. "Nixon Started the War on Drugs. Privately, He Said Pot Was 'Not Particularly Dangerous,'" *New York Times*, Sept. 14, 2024, nytimes.com/2024/09/14/us/nixon-marijuana-tapes.html.

3 ACLU. "The War on Marijuana in Black and White," June 3, 2013, aclu.org/the-war-on-marijuana-in-black-and-white.

4 Jaeger, Kyle. "9 in 10 Americans Support Legalizing Marijuana in Some Form, Including Bipartisan Majorities, Pew Poll Shows," *Marijuana Moment*, July 8, 2025, tinyurl.com/3n4a2b7k.

5 Harrar, Sari. "Medical Marijuana: Your Questions Answered and What We Know Today," AARP, Sept. 3, 2019, tinyurl.com/yc8hrpn2.

6 Nania, Rachel. "1 in 5 Older Adults Uses Cannabis," AARP, Sept. 12, 2024, tinyurl.com/vp49j25r.

7 Nania, Rachel. "Marijuana Use Among Older Adults Climbs to New High," AARP, June 3, 2025, aarp.org/health/drugs-supplements/rising-marijuana-use-in-older-adults.html.

8 Kaskie, B. et al. "Unrelenting Growth and Diversification: Using the Health and Retirement Study to Illuminate Cannabis Use Among Aging Americans," *Gerontologist* 64(6) (June 2024), doi.org/10.1093/geront/gnae016.

9 Lent, Michelle R. et al. "Changes in Health-Related Quality of Life over the First Three Months of Medical Marijuana Use," *Journal of Cannabis Research* 64(6), S. 2 (Sept. 11, 2024), tinyurl.com/5ea5mmyp; Arkell, Thomas R. et al. "Assessment of Medical Cannabis and Health-Related Quality of Life," *JAMA Network Open* 6(5):e2312522 (2023). doi.org/10.1001/jamanetworkopen.2023.12522.

10 Singh, Gurkirpal. "Recent Considerations in Nonsteroidal Anti-Inflammatory Drug Gastropathy," *American Journal of Medicine* 105(1), S. 2 (July 27, 1998), sciencedirect.com/science/article/pii/S0002934398000722.

11 Abuhasira, Ran et al. "Epidemiological Characteristics, Safety and Efficacy of Medical Cannabis in the Elderly," *European Journal of Internal Medicine* 49 (March 2018), doi.org/10.1016/j.ejim.2018.01.019.

12 Mokrysz, Claire et al. "Are IQ and Educational Outcomes in Teenagers Related to Their Cannabis Use? A Prospective Cohort Study," *Journal of Psychopharmacology* 30(2) (Feb. 2016), doi.org/10.1177/0269881115622241.

13 Callaghan, Russell C. et al. "Cannabis Use and Incidence of Testicular Cancer: A 42-Year Follow-Up of Swedish Men Between 1970 and 2011," *Cancer Epidemiology, Biomarkers & Prevention* 26(11) (Nov. 2017), doi.org/10.1158/1055-9965.EPI-17-0428.

14 Li, Xuan Xuan et al. "The Global Burden of Schizophrenia and the Impact of Urbanization During 1990–2019: An Analysis of the Global Burden of Disease Study 2019," *Environmental Research* 232 (Sept. 1, 2023), doi.org/10.1016/j.envres.2023.116305; "Alcohol, Drugs and Addictive Behaviours: Cannabis," World Health Organization, accessed Aug. 20, 2025, who.int/teams/mental-health-and-substance-use/alcohol-drugs-and-addictive-behaviours/drugs-psychoactive/cannabis.

15 Gruber, S. A. et al. "The Grass Might Be Greener: Medical Marijuana Patients Exhibit Altered Brain Activity and Improved Executive Function after 3 Months of Treatment," *Frontiers in Pharmacology* 8 (Jan. 16, 2018), doi.org/10.3389/fphar.2017.00983.

16 Payne, Kelly S. et al. "Cannabis and Male Fertility: A Systematic Review," *Journal of Urology* 202(4) (Sep. 6, 2019), doi.org/10.1097/JU.0000000000000248.

**Chapter 2: What Is Cannabis and How Is It Used?**

1 Tashkin, Donald P. "Marijuana and Lung Disease," *Chest* 154(3) (Sept. 2018), doi.org/10.1016/j.chest.2018.05.005.

2 Dahlgren, M. K. et al. "A Survey-Based, Quasi-Experimental Study Assessing a High-Cannabidiol Suppository for Menstrual-Related Pain and Discomfort," *npj Women's Health* 2(29) (2024), doi.org/10.1038/s44294-024-00032-0.

3 Guggisberg, J. et al. "Cannabis as an Anticancer Agent: A Review of Clinical Data and Assessment of Case Reports," *Cannabis and Cannabinoid Research* 7(1) (Feb. 2022), doi.org/10.1089/can.2021.0045.

**Chapter 3: Aging Isn't for the Faint of Heart**

1 Walker, M. et al. "Age-Related Patterns of Medical Cannabis Use: A Survey of Authorized Patients in Canada," *Cannabis* 7(2) (June 26, 2024): 135, doi.org/10.26828/cannabis/2024/000208.

**Chapter 4: How Can Cannabis Help?**

1 Abuhasira, Ran et al. "Epidemiological Characteristics, Safety and Efficacy of Medical Cannabis in the Elderly," *European Journal of Internal Medicine* 49 (Mar. 2018): 44, doi.org/10.1016/j.ejim.2018.01.019.

2 Abuhasira, Ran et al. "Medical Cannabis for Older Patients—Treatment Protocol and Initial Results," *Journal of Clinical Medicine* 8(11) (Nov. 1, 2019), doi.org/10.3390/jcm8111819.

3 Walker, M. et al. "Age-related Patterns of Medical Cannabis Use: A Survey of Authorized Patients in Canada," *Cannabis* 7(2) (June 26, 2024): 135–149, 135, doi.org/10.26828/cannabis/2024/000208.

4 National Academies of Sciences, Engineering, and Medicine. *The Health Effects of Cannabis and Cannabinoids: The Current State of Evidence and Recommendations for Research* (Washington, DC: National Academies Press, 2017), 88, doi.org/10.17226/24625.

5 Sagy, Iftach et al. "Safety and Efficacy of Medical Cannabis in Fibromyalgia," *Journal of Clinical Medicine* 8(6) (June 5, 2019), doi.org/10.3390/jcm8060807.

6 Singla, Abhinav A. et al. "A Cross-Sectional Survey Study of Cannabis Use for Fibromyalgia Symptom Management," *Mayo Clinic Proceedings* 99(4) (Apr. 2024): 542–550, 542, doi.org/10.1016/j.mayocp.2023.12.018.

7 Spindle, T. R. et al. "Vaporized D-Limonene Selectively Mitigates the Acute Anxiogenic Effects of Δ9-Tetrahydrocannabinol in Healthy Adults Who Intermittently Use Cannabis," *Drug and Alcohol Dependence* 257 (Apr. 1, 2024), doi.org/10.1016/j.drugalcdep.2024.111267.

8 Drake, C. et al. "Medical Cannabis Availability and Mental Health: Evidence from New York's Medical Cannabis Program," National Bureau of Economic Research, Working Paper Series (May 2024), doi.org/10.3386/w32514. nber.org/papers/w32514.

9 Lynskey, M. T. et al. "Prescribed Medical Cannabis Use Among Older Individuals: Patient Characteristics and Improvements in Well-Being: Findings from T21," *Drugs and Aging* 41(6) (June 2024): 521–530, doi.org/10.1007/s40266-024-01123-y.

10 Bonn-Miller, Marcel O. et al. "The Long-Term, Prospective, Therapeutic Impact of Cannabis on Post-Traumatic Stress Disorder," *Cannabis and Cannabinoid Research* 7(2) (Apr. 2022): 214–223, 214, doi.org/10.1089/can.2020.0056.

11 Lynskey et al. "Prescribed Medical Cannabis Use Among Older Individuals."

12 Megelin, Thomas and Ghorayeb, Imad. "Cannabis for Restless Legs Syndrome: A Report of Six Patients," *Sleep Medicine* 36 (2017): 182, doi.org/10.1016/j.sleep.2017.04.019.

13 Otman, Haley. "More People with MS Turning to Cannabis for Help with Pain, Sleep," *Michigan Medicine*, Univ. of Michigan, Feb. 15, 2021, tinyurl.com/3bfxz9uv.

14 Russo, Margherita et al., "Sativex in the Management of Multiple Sclerosis-Related Spasticity: Role of the Corticospinal Modulation," *Neural Plasticity* 2015 (Jan. 9, 2015), doi.org/10.1155/2015/656582.

15 Torri Clerici, Valentina et al., "Nabiximols Oromucosal Spray in Patients with Multiple Sclerosis-Related Bladder Dysfunction: A Prospective Study," *Multiple Sclerosis and Related Disorders* 74 (June 2023), doi.org/10.1016/j.msard.2023.104711.

16 Dolhun, Rachel. "MJFF Survery Results: People with Parkinson's Share Experiences with Cannabis," Michael J. Fox Foundation, Jan. 21, 2022, tinyurl.com/mry6wz66.

17 Ruver-Martins, Ana Carolina et al. "Low Doses of Cannabis Extract Ameliorate Non-Motor Symptoms of Parkinson's Disease Patients: A Case Series," *Frontiers in Human Neuroscience* 18 (Feb. 23, 2025), doi.org/10.3389/fnhum.2024.1466438.

18 Goldberg, Tomer et al. "Long-Term Safety of Medical Cannabis in Parkinson's Disease: A Retrospective Case-Control Study," *Parkinsonism and Related Disorders* 112 (July 2023), doi.org/10.1016/j.parkreldis.2023.105406.

19 Akinyemi, Edward et al. "Medical Marijuana Effects in Movement Disorders, Focus on Huntington Disease; A Literature Review," *Journal of Pharmacy & Pharmaceutical Sciences* 23 (2020), doi.org/10.18433/jpps30967.

20 National Academies of Sciences, Engineering, and Medicine. *The Health Effects of Cannabis and Cannabinoids: The Current State of Evidence and Recommendations for Research* (National Academies Press, 2017), doi.org/10.17226/24625; Bathula, Pavana P. and Mciver, M. Bruce. "Cannabinoids in Treating Chemotherapy-Induced Nausea and Vomiting, Cancer-Associated Pain, and Tumor Growth," *International Journal of Molecular Sciences* 25(1) (Dec. 20, 2023), doi.org/10.3390/ijms25010074; Tramèr, Martin R. et al. "Cannabinoids for Chemotherapy Induced Nausea and Vomiting: Quantitative Systematic Review," *BMJ: British Medical Journal* 323(7303) (July 7, 2001), doi.org/10.1136/bmj.323.7303.16.

21 Fahey, Margaret C. et al. "Cannabis Perceptions and Patterns of Use Among Older Adult Cancer Survivors," *Journal of Aging and Health* 37(1–2) (Jan. 2025), doi.org/10.1177/08982643241231320.

22 Russo, Ethan B. "Clinical Endocannabinoid Deficiency Reconsidered: Current Research Supports the Theory in Migraine, Fibromyalgia, Irritable Bowel, and Other Treatment-Resistant Syndromes," *Cannabis and Cannabinoid Research* 1(1) (July 1, 2016): 154–165, doi.org/10.1089/can.2016.0009.

23 Desai, Parth et al. "Association Between Cannabis Use and Healthcare Utilization in Patients With Irritable Bowel Syndrome: A Retrospective Cohort Study," *Cureus: Journal of Medical Science* 12(5) (May 7, 2020), doi.org/10.7759/cureus.8008.

24 Kogilathota, J. et al. "Impact of Cannabis Use in Patients with Inflammatory Bowel Disease: Insights from the National Readmission Database 2019-2020," *American Journal of Gastroenterology* 119(10S) (Oct. 2024): S771, doi.org/10.14309/01.ajg.0001033716.68359.b3.

25 Naftali, T. et al. "Oral CBD-Rich Cannabis Induces Clinical but Not Endoscopic Response in Patients with Crohn's Disease, a Randomised Controlled Trial," *Journal of Crohn's and Colitis* 15(11) (2021): 1799–1806, doi.org/10.1093/ecco-jcc/jjab069.

26 Abdel-Salam, O. "Gastric Acid Inhibitory and Gastric Protective Effects of Cannabis and Cannabinoids," *Asian Pacific Journal of Tropical Medicine* 9 (May 2016), doi.org/10.1016/j.apjtm.2016.04.021.

27 Blake D. R. et al. "Preliminary Assessment of the Efficacy, Tolerability, and Safety of a Cannabis-Based Medicine (Sativex) in the Treatment of Pain Caused by Rheumatoid Arthritis," *Rheumatology* 45(1) (Jan. 2006): 50–52, doi.org/10.1093/rheumatology/kei183.

28 Ceolin, C. et al. "The Potential of Cannabinoids in Managing Cancer-Related Anorexia in Older Adults: A Systematic Review of the Literature," *The Journal of Nutrition, Health and Aging* 28(8) (Aug. 2024), doi.org/10.1016/j.jnha.2024.100299.

29 Cyr, C. et al. "Cannabis in Palliative Care: Current Challenges and Practical Recommendations." *Annals of Palliative Medicine* 7(4) (Oct. 2018): 463–477, doi.org/10.21037/apm.2018.06.04.

30 Streicher, L. "Use and Perceived Impact of Cannabis on Orgasm in Post Menopause Women," *Journal of Sexual Medicine* 21 (S. 5) (June 2024): qdae054.020, doi.org/10.1093/jsxmed/qdae054.020.

31 Silva, E. A. D. et al. "Cannabis and Cannabinoid Use in Autism Spectrum Disorder: A Systematic Review," *Trends in Psychiatry and Psychotherapy* (June 13, 2022): e20200149, doi.org/10.47626/2237-6089-2020-0149.

32 Riva, N. et al. "Safety and Efficacy of Nabiximols on Spasticity Symptoms in Patients with Motor Neuron Disease (CANALS): A Multicentre, Double-Blind, Randomised, Placebo-Controlled, Phase 2 Trial," *Lancet Neurology* 18(2) (Feb. 2019): 155–164, doi.org/10.1016/S1474-4422(18)30406-X.

33 Denton, T. T. et al. "Amyotrophic Lateral Sclerosis, the Endocannabinoid System, and Exogenous Cannabinoids: Current State and Clinical Implications," *Muscle & Nerve* 72(1) (July 2025): 7–14, doi.org/10.1002/mus.28359.

34 Bahji, A. et al. "Cannabinoids in the Management of Behavioral, Psychological, and Motor Symptoms of Neurocognitive Disorders: A Mixed Studies Systematic Review," *Journal of Cannabis Research* 4(11) (March 2022), doi.org/10.1186/s42238-022-00119-y.

35 Herrmann, N. et al. "Randomized Placebo-Controlled Trial of Nabilone for Agitation in Alzheimer's Disease," *American Journal of Geriatric Psychiatry* 27(11) (Nov. 2019): 1161–1173, doi.org/10.1016/j.jagp.2019.05.002.

36 Navarro, Cristian E., and Pérez, Juan C. "Treatment of Neuropsychiatric Symptoms in Alzheimer's Disease with a Cannabis-Based Magistral Formulation: An Open-Label Prospective Cohort Study," *Medical Cannabis and Cannabinoids* 7(1) (Sept. 12, 2024): 160–170, doi.org/10.1159/000541364.

37 Pessoa, R. M. P. et al., "Effects of Cannabidiol on Behavioral and Psychological Symptoms of Vascular Dementia: A Randomized, Double-Blind, Placebo-Controlled Trial," *International Psychogeriatrics* 36, S. 1 (Sept. 2024): 132–133, doi.org/10.1017/S1041610224002588.

38 Myran, D. T. et al. "Risk of Dementia in Individuals with Emergency Department Visits or Hospitalizations Due to Cannabis," *JAMA Neurology* 82(6) (June 1, 2025): 570–579, doi.org/10.1001/jamaneurol.2025.0530.

39 Osler, William. *The Principles and Practices of Medicine* (Edinburgh and London: Young J. Putland, 1892), loc.gov/item/03000585/.

40 Avila, Christina et al. "Cannabinoids for the Treatment of Chronic Pruritus: A Review," *Journal of the American Academy of Dermatology* 82(5) (May 2020): 1205–1212, jaad.org/article/S0190-9622(20)30120-1/abstract.

41 Kuzumi, A. et al. "The Potential Role of Cannabidiol in Cosmetic Dermatology: A Literature Review," *American Journal of Clinical Dermatology* 25(6) (Nov. 2024): 951–966, doi.org/10.1007/s40257-024-00891-y.

42 Grinspoon, Lester. *Marihuana Reconsidered: The Most Thorough Evaluation of the Benefits & Dangers of Cannabis* (Cambridge, MA: Harvard Univ. Press, 1971).

43 Li, L. and Deng, Q. C. "Loneliness and Cannabis Use Among Older Adults: Findings from a Canada National Survey During the Covid-19 Pandemic," *BMC Public Health* 24(1) (Oct. 28, 2024): 2983, doi.org/10.1186/s12889-024-20499-5.

44 Ibid.

45 Lynskey. "Prescribed Medical Cannabis Use among Older Individuals."

46 Gruber, Staci A. et al. "The Grass Might Be Greener: Medical Marijuana Patients Exhibit Altered Brain Activity and Improved Executive Function after 3 Months of Treatment," *Frontiers in Pharmacology* 8 (Jan. 16, 2018), doi.org/10.3389/fphar.2017.00983.

47 Stringer, Heather. "Reclassification of Cannabis Is a Win for Researchers," American Psychological Association, June 11, 2024, apa.org/topics/substance-use-abuse-addiction/cannabis-reclassification-researchers.

48 Thurgur, H. et al. "Cannabis-Based Medicinal Products (CBMPs) for the Treatment of Long COVID Symptoms: Current and Potential Applications," *Exploration of Medicine* 4 (2023): 487–503, doi.org/10.37349/emed.2023.00158.

**Chapter 5: Potential Harms of Cannabis for Older Patients (and Others)**

1 Dvorak, R. D. et al. "Effects of Medical Cannabis Use on Physical and Psychiatric Symptoms Across the Day Among Older Adults," *Psychiatry Research* 339 (Sept. 2024): 116055, doi.org/10.1016/j.psychres.2024.116055.

2 Curfman, Gregory. "FDA Strengthens Warning that NSAIDs Increase Heart Attack and Stroke Risk," Harvard Health Publishing, June 25, 2019, health.harvard.edu/blog/fda-strengthens-warning-that-nsaids-increase-heart-attack-and-stroke-risk-201507138138.

3 Jeffers, A. M. et al. "Association of Cannabis Use with Cardiovascular Outcomes Among US Adults," *Journal of the American Heart Association* 13(5) (Mar. 5, 2024): e030178, doi.org/10.1161/JAHA.123.030178.

4 van Amsterdam, J., and van den Brink, W. "Cannabis Use Variations and Myocardial Infarction: A Systematic Review," *Journal of Clinical Medicine* 13(18) (Sept. 22, 2024): 5620, doi.org/10.3390/jcm13185620.

5 American Heart Association News. "Marijuana Use Linked to Higher Risk of Heart Attack and Stroke," Feb. 28, 2024, tinyurl.com/2skckufs.

6 Sebastian, S. A. et al. "Cannabis Use and Atherosclerotic Cardiovascular Disease Outcomes: A Meta-Analysis of Multinational Cohort Data," *Disease-a-Month* 71(3) (2025), doi.org/10.1016/j.disamonth.2024.101849.

7 Kamel, I. et al. "Myocardial Infarction and Cardiovascular Risks Associated with Cannabis Use: A Multicenter Retrospective Study," *JACC Advances* 4(5) (May 2025), doi.org/10.1016/j.jacadv.2025.101698.

8 Tashkin, D. P. and Tan, W. C. "Inhaled Marijuana and the Lung," *Journal of Allergy and Clinical Immunology: In Practice* 10(11) (Nov. 2022): 2822–2829, doi.org/10.1016/j.jaip.2022.05.009.

9 CDC Archive. "Tobacco-Related Mortality" (2020), archive.cdc.gov/www_cdc_gov/tobacco/data_statistics/fact_sheets/health_effects/tobacco_related_mortality/index.htm; Melamede, Robert. "Cannabis and Tobacco Smoke Are Not Equally Carcinogenic," *Harm Reduction Journal* 2(21) (Oct. 18, 2005), doi.org/10.1186/1477-7517-2-21.

10 Malesu, Vijay Kumar. "Older Drivers Show Evidence of Impaired Driving Performance after Smoking Cannabis, Even If They Regularly Usa Cannabis," *News-Medical*, Jan. 22, 2024, tinyurl.com/4wezv7k2.

11 Meda, S. A. et al. "A Randomized, Placebo-Controlled, Double-Blind, Pilot Study of Cannabis-Related Driving Impairment Assessed by Driving Simulator and Self-Report." *Journal of Psychopharmacology* 39(4) (Apr. 2025): 364–372, doi.org/10.1177/02698811251324379.

12 Smith, R. T. and Gruber, S. A. "Contemplating Cannabis? The Complex Relationship Between Cannabinoids and Hepatic Metabolism Resulting in the Potential for Drug–Drug Interactions," *Frontiers in Psychiatry* 13 (Jan. 10, 2023): 1055481, doi.org/10.3389/fpsyt.2022.1055481.

13 Nachnani, R. et al. (2024). "Systematic Review of Drug–Drug Interactions of Delta-9-Tetrahydrocannabinol, Cannabidiol, and Cannabis," *Frontiers in Pharmacology* 15 (May 22, 2024): 1282831, doi.org/10.3389/fphar.2024.1282831.

14 So, G. C. et al. "A Phase I Trial of the Pharmacokinetic Interaction Between Cannabidiol and Tacrolimus," *Clinical Pharmacology & Therapeutics* 117(3) (Mar. 2025): 716–723, doi.org/10.1002/cpt.3504.

15 Alexander, J. C. and Joshi, G.P. "A Review of the Anesthetic Implications of Marijuana Use," *Baylor University Medical Center Proceedings* 32(3) (May 21, 2019): 364–371, doi.org/10.1080/08998280.2019.1603034.

16 Myran, D. T. et al. "Risk of Dementia in Individuals with Emergency Department Visits or Hospitalizations Due to Cannabis," *JAMA Neurology* 82(6) (June 1, 2025): 570–579, doi.org/10.1001/jamaneurol.2025.0530.

17 Nield, David. "Cannabis Revealed to Have Anti-Aging Effect in the Brains of Mice," *Science Alert*, Aug. 26, 2024, tinyurl.com/bdumcxp6.

18 Høeg, K. M. et al. "Cannabis Use and Age-Related Changes in Cognitive Function from Early Adulthood to Late Midlife in 5162 Danish Men," *Brain and Behavior* 14 (Nov. 2024): e70136, doi.org/10.1002/brb3.70136.

19 Fernández-Ruiz, Javier. "Cannabidiol for Neurodegenerative Disorders: Important New Clinical Applications for this Phytocannabinoid?" *British Journal of Clinical Pharmacology* 75(2) (May 25, 2012): 323–333, doi.org/10.1111/j.1365-2125.2012.04341.x.

20 Workman, C. D. et al. "Increased Likelihood of Falling in Older Cannabis Users vs. Non-Users," *Brain Sciences* 11(2) (Jan. 21, 2021): 134, doi.org/10.3390/brainsci11020134.

21 Bab, K. M. et al. "Detection of Ethanol, Cannabinoids, Benzodiazepines, and Opioids in Older Adults Evaluated for Serious Injuries from Falls," *Clinical Toxicology* 62(10) (Oct. 2024): 661–668, doi.org/10.1080/15563650.2024.2400186.

22 Leung, Miriam T. Y. "Gabapentinoids and Risk of Hip Fracture," *JAMA Network* 7(11) (Nov. 13, 2024): e2444488, doi.org/10.1001/jamanetworkopen.2024.44488.

23 Abuhasira, Ran et al. "Epidemiological Characteristics, Safety and Efficacy of Medical Cannabis in the Elderly," *European Journal of Internal Medicine* 49 (Mar. 2018): 44–50, doi.org/10.1016/j.ejim.2018.01.019.

24 Han, B. H. et al. "Trends in Emergency Department Visits Associated with Cannabis Use Among Older Adults in California, 2005–2019," *Journal of the American Geriatrics Society* 71(4) (Apr. 2023): 1267–1274, doi.org/10.1111/jgs.18180.

### Chapter 6: What Are the Practicalities of Using Medical Cannabis?

1 Piomelli, D. and Russo, E. B. "The *Cannabis Sativa* Versus *Cannabis Indica* Debate: An Interview with Ethan Russo, MD," *Cannabis and Cannabinoid Research* 1(1) (Jan. 1, 2016): 44–46, doi.org/10.1089/can.2015.29003.

2 "Racial Disparity in Marijuana Arrests," NORML Fact Sheet, n.d., norml.org/marijuana/fact-sheets/racial-disparity-in-marijuana-arrests/.

3 French, M. T. et al. "The Relationships Between Marijuana Use and Exercise Among Young and Middle-Aged Adults," *Preventive Medicine* 147 (June 2021): 106518, doi.org/10.1016/j.ypmed.2021.106518.

4 Dahlke, S. et al. "The Effects of Stigma: Older Persons and Medicinal Cannabis," *Qualitative Health Research* 34(8–9) (July 2024): 717–731, doi.org/10.1177/10497323241227419.

5 Grinspoon, Peter. *Seeing Through the Smoke: A Cannabis Specialist Untangles the Truth About Marijuana* (Lanham, MD: Prometheus, 2023).

### Chapter 7: What Role Does CBD Play in Addressing Health Issues as We Age?

1 Weiner, Stacy. "CBD: Does it Work? Is it Safe? Is it Legal?" AAMC, July 20, 2023, tinyurl.com/4bcxbtzt.

2 Choi, N. G. et al. "Cannabidiol Use Among Older Adults: Associations with Cannabis Use, Physical and Mental Health, and Other Substance Use," *Clinical Gerontologist* (Nov. 22, 2024): 1–13, doi.org/10.1080/07317115.2024.2429595.

3 Porter, B. et al. "Cannabidiol (CBD) Use by Older Adults for Acute and Chronic Pain," *Journal of Gerontological Nursing* 47(7) (July 2021): 6–15, doi.org/10.3928/00989134-20210610-02.

4 Bhaskar, A. et al. (2021). "Consensus Recommendations on Dosing and Administration of Medical Cannabis to Treat Chronic Pain: Results of a Modified Delphi Process," *Journal of Cannabis Research* 3(22) (2021), doi.org/10.1186/s42238-021-00073-1.

5 Arnold, J. C. et al. "The Safety and Efficacy of Low Oral Doses of Cannabidiol: An Evaluation of the Evidence," *Clinical and Translational Science* 16(1) (Jan. 2023): 10–30, doi.org/10.1111/cts.13425.

6 So, G. C. et al. "A Phase I Trial of the Pharmacokinetic Interaction Between Cannabidiol and Tacrolimus," *Clinical Pharmacology & Therapeutics* 117 (Nov. 2024): 716–723, doi.org/10.1002/cpt.3504.

7 Tumati, S. et al. "Medical Cannabis Use Among Older Adults in Canada: Self-Reported Data on Types and Amount Used, and Perceived Effects," *Drugs and Aging* 39(2) (Feb. 2022): 153–163, doi.org/10.1007/s40266-021-00913-y.

8 Bergamaschi, M. M. et al. "Cannabidiol Reduces the Anxiety Induced by Simulated Public Speaking in Treatment-Naïve Social Phobia Patients," *Neuropsychopharmacology* 36(6) (May 2011): 1219–1226, doi.org/10.1038/npp.2011.6.

9 Coelho, C. F. et al. "The Impact of Cannabidiol Treatment on Anxiety Disorders: A Systematic Review of Randomized Controlled Clinical Trials," *Life* (Basel) 14(11) (Oct. 25, 2024): 1373, doi.org/10.3390/life14111373.

10 Ozonsi, R. et al. "Caring for Behavioral Symptoms of Dementia (CBD): A New Investigation into Cannabidiol for the Treatment of Anxiety and Agitation in Alzheimer's Dementia," *American Journal of Geriatric Psychiatry* 32, S. 4 (2024), doi.org/10.1016/j.jagp.2024.01.172.

11 Leszko, M. (2023). "Use of Cannabidiol Oil by Caregivers: A Focus on Alzheimer's Disease," *Medicinal Use of Cannabis and Cannabinoids* (2023): 129–134, doi.org/10.1016/B978-0-323-90036-2.00045-4.

12 Mohammed, Sherin Yasser Mostafa et al. "Effectiveness of Cannabidiol to Manage Chronic Pain: A Systematic Review," *Pain Management Nursing* 25(2) (Apr. 2024): e76–e86, doi.org/10.1016/j.pmn.2023.10.002.

13 Cásedas, G. et al. "Cannabidiol (CBD): A Systematic Review of Clinical and Preclinical Evidence in the Treatment of Pain," *Pharmaceuticals* (Basel) 17(11) (Oct. 28, 2024): 1438, doi.org/10.3390/ph17111438.

14 Ranum, R. M. et al. "Use of Cannabidiol in the Management of Insomnia: A Systematic Review," *Cannabis and Cannabinoid Research* 8(2) (Apr. 2023): 213–229, doi.org/10.1089/can.2022.0122.

15 Strickland, J. C. et al. "Cross-Sectional and Longitudinal Evaluation of Cannabidiol (CBD) Product Use and Health Among People with Epilepsy," *Epilepsy & Behavior* 122 (Sept. 2021): 108205, doi.org/10.1016/j.yebeh.2021.108205.

16 de Oliveira, V. G. et al. "The Efficacy of Cannabidiol for Seizures Reduction in Pharmacoresistant Epilepsy: A Systematic Review and Meta-Analysis," *Acta Epileptologica* 7(1) (Mar. 17, 2025): 20, doi.org/10.1186/s42494-024-00191-2.

17 Batalla, A. et al. "The Potential of Cannabidiol as a Treatment for Psychosis and Addiction: Who Benefits Most? A Systematic Review," *Journal of Clinical Medicine* 8(7) (July 19, 2019): 1058, doi.org/10.3390/jcm8071058.

18 Englund, Amir et al. "Cannabidiol Inhibits THC-Elicited Paranoid Symptoms and Hippocampal-Dependent Memory Impairment," *Journal of Psychopharmacology* 27(1) (Oct. 5, 2012): 19–27, doi.org/10.1177/0269881112460109.

19 Hindocha, C. et al. "Cannabidiol Reverses Attentional Bias to Cigarette Cues in a Human Experimental Model of Tobacco Withdrawal," *Addiction* 113(9) (May 1, 2018): 1696–1705, doi.org/10.1111/add.14243.

20 Hurd, Y. L. et al. "Cannabidiol for the Reduction of Cue-Induced Craving and Anxiety in Drug-Abstinent Individuals with Heroin Use Disorder: A Double-Blind Randomized Placebo-Controlled Trial," *American Journal of Psychiatry* 176(11) (Nov. 1, 2019): 911–922, doi.org/10.1176/appi.ajp.2019.18101191. Erratum in: *American Journal of Psychiatry* 177(7) (July 1, 2020): 641, doi.org/10.1176/appi.ajp.2020.18101191correction.

21 Mosslett, Marie. "CDB and CBG Ointment Improved Skin in Patients with Atopic Dermatitis," *Dermatology Times*, Mar. 26, 2025, tinyurl.com/26j5kd35.

22 Grinspoon, Lester. "The NFL Should Combat Concussions with Cannabis," *Vice*, Feb. 27, 2014, tinyurl.com/mecapka9.

23 McCartney, D. et al. "Effects of Cannabidiol on Simulated Driving and Cognitive Performance: A Dose-Ranging Randomised Controlled Trial," *Journal of Psychopharmacology* 36(12) (Dec. 2022): 1338–1349, doi.org/10.1177/02698811221095356.

24 Cuttler, C. et al. "Acute Effects of Cannabigerol on Anxiety, Stress, and Mood: A Double-Blind, Placebo-Controlled, Crossover, Field Trial," *Scientific Reports* 14(1) (July 13, 2024): 16163, doi.org/10.1038/s41598-024-66879-0.

### Chapter 8: Beyond the Medicinal: Lifestyle Improvements for Older Patients

1 Mulvehill, S. and Tishler, J. "Assessment of the Effect of Cannabis Use Before Partnered Sex on Women with and Without Orgasm Difficulty," *The Journal of Sexual Medicine* 12(2) (May 6, 2024): qfae023, doi.org/10.1093/sexmed/qfae023.

2 Banbury, S. et al. "A Preliminary Investigation into the Use of Cannabis Suppositories and Online Mindful Compassion for Improving Sexual Function Among Women Following Gynaecological Cancer Treatment," *Medicina* (Kaunas) 60(12) (Dec. 7, 2024): 2020, doi.org/10.3390/medicina60122020.

3 Sagan, Carl. "Acute Intoxication: Literary Reports—Mr. X," Library of Consciousness, 1969, organism.earth/library/document/mr-x.

4 Boutouis, S. et al. "The Association between Marijuana and E-Cigarette Use and Exercise Behavior Among Adults," *Preventive Medicine Reports* 40 (Feb. 28, 2024): 102668, doi.org/10.1016/j.pmedr.2024.102668.

5 Sagan. "Acute Intoxication."

6 Sagan, Carl. *The Dragons of Eden: Speculations on the Evolution of Human* (New York: Ballantine, 1986).

7 Tart, Charles T. *On Being Stoned: A Psychological Study of Marijuana Intoxication* (Palo Alto, CA: Science and Behavior Books, 1971), chap. 4.

8 Ibid., chap. 15.

9 National Institute on Alcohol Abuse and Alcoholism. "Alcohol-Related Emergencies and Deaths in the United States," National Institutes of Health, Nov. 2024, niaaa .nih.gov/alcohols-effects-health/alcohol-topics-z/alcohol-facts-and-statistics /alcohol-related-emergencies-and-deaths-united-states.

### Chapter 9: How Psychedelic Drugs Might Help

1 Serafini, G. et al. "The Role of Ketamine in Treatment-Resistant Depression: A Systematic Review," *Current Neuropharmacology* 12(5) (Sep. 2014): 444–461, doi.org/10.2174/1570159X12666140619204251.

2 Bogenschutz, M. P. et al. "Percentage of Heavy Drinking Days Following Psilocybin-Assisted Psychotherapy vs Placebo in the Treatment of Adult Patients with Alcohol Use Disorder: A Randomized Clinical Trial," *JAMA Psychiatry* 79(10) (2022): 953–962. doi.org/10.1001/jamapsychiatry.2022.2096.

3 McDonnell, R. et al. "AA, Bill Wilson, Carl Jung and LSD," *Analytical Psychology* 69(4) (July 30, 2024): 550–580, doi.org/10.1111/1468-5922.13027.

4 Collins, H. M. "Psychedelics for the Treatment of Obsessive-Compulsive Disorder: Efficacy and Proposed Mechanisms," *International Journal of Neuropsychopharmacology* 27(12) (Dec. 1, 2024): pyae057, doi.org/10.1093/ijnp/pyae057.

5 Riaz, K. et al. "MDMA-Based Psychotherapy in Treatment-Resistant Post-Traumatic Stress Disorder (PTSD): A Brief Narrative Overview of Current Evidence," *Diseases* 11(4) (Nov. 3, 2023): 159, doi.org/10.3390/diseases11040159.

6 Jacobs, Andrew. "'Life-Changing' Psychedelics, for When Life Is Ending," *New York Times*, Dec. 17, 2024, tinyurl.com/msf39mc5.

7 Cornish, N. et al. "Psychedelics, Spirituality, and Existential Distress in Patients at the End of Life," *Cleveland Clinic Journal of Medicine* 92(4) (Apr. 2025): 248–254, doi.org/10.3949/ccjm.92a.24100.

8 Marchi, M. et al. "Psychedelics as an Intervention for Psychological, Existential Distress in Terminally Ill Patients: A Systematic Review and Network Meta-Analysis," *Journal of Psychopharmacology* (Dec. 10, 2024): 2698811241303594, doi.org/10.1177/02698811241303594.

9 Griffiths, R. R. et al. "Psilocybin Produces Substantial and Sustained Decreases in Depression and Anxiety in Patients with Life-Threatening Cancer: A Randomized Double-Blind Trial," *Journal of Psychopharmacology* 30(12) (Dec. 2016): 1181–1197, doi.org/10.1177/0269881116675513.

10 Agin-Liebes, G. I. et al. "Long-Term Follow-Up of Psilocybin-Assisted Psychotherapy for Psychiatric and Existential Distress in Patients with Life-Threatening Cancer," *Journal of Psychopharmacology* 34(2) (Feb. 2020): 155–166, doi.org/10.1177/0269881119897615.

11 de Quevedo, Joao L. "FDA Grants Breakthrough Status to LSD Formula and Opens a New Frontier in the Generalized Anxiety Disorder (GAD) Treatment," McGovern Medical School, Apr. 1, 2024, tinyurl.com/4ea5cyfh.

12 "Statement from National Council of Native American Churches and the Indigenous Peyote Conservation Initiative Regarding Decriminalization of Sacred Plants . . . as They Pertain to Peyote." 2020, tinyurl.com/tddykas9; Sahugún, Louis. "Why Are Some Native Americans Fighting Efforts to Decriminalize Peyote?" *Los Angeles Times*, Mar. 29, 2020, tinyurl.com/2rx4x2ff.

13 Dolan, Eric W. "Study: 'Bad Trips' from Magic Mushrooms Often Result in an Improved Sense of Personal Well-Being," *PsyPost*, Aug. 30, 2016, tinyurl.com/wyxcd7yz.

## Afterword

1 St. Pierre, Allen. "America's 20-Millionth Marijuana Arrest—Coming to Your Home or Person?" NORML, Oct. 3, 2008, norml.org/blog/2008/10/03/americas-20-millionth-marijuana-arrest-coming-to-your-home-or-person/.

# Index

Note: Italicized page numbers indicate images.

# About the Author

**Peter Grinspoon, MD,** is a primary care physician and cannabis specialist at Massachusetts General Hospital and an instructor in medicine at Harvard Medical School. He is also a certified addiction medicine specialist, and a certified health and wellness coach. Dr. Grinspoon is a board member of the advocacy group Doctors for Drug Policy Reform and an advisor to the Parabola Group, which advocates for social justice in the cannabis space. He spent two years as an associate director of the Massachusetts Physician Health Service, treating and monitoring hundreds of physicians with addiction. He is the author of the memoir *Free Refills: A Doctor Confronts His Addiction*. Dr. Grinspoon is a widely recognized expert on cannabis science and drug policy and is a contributing editor to Harvard Health Publishing. He has been on NPR's *All Things Considered*, as well as national television shows including *NBC Nightly News* and MSNBC.